LECTURES
HISTORY OF P

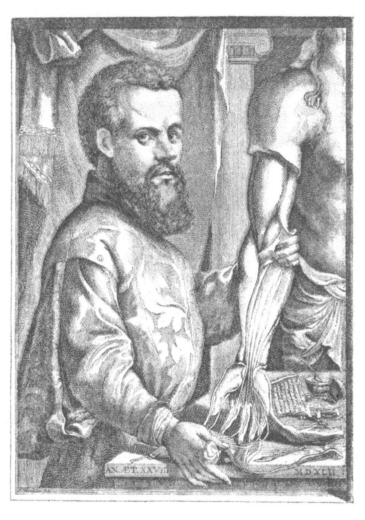

ANDREAS VESALIUS

BRUXELLENSIS, SCHOLAE MEDICORUM PATAVINAE PROFESSOR

LECTURES ON THE HISTORY OF PHYSIOLOGY

DURING THE SIXTEENTH, SEVEN-TEENTH AND EIGHTEENTH CENTURIES

BY

SIR MICHAEL FOSTER

CAMBRIDGE
AT THE UNIVERSITY PRESS
1924

CAMBRIDGE UNIVERSITY PRESS
Cambridge, New York, Melbourne, Madrid, Cape Town,
Singapore, São Paulo, Delhi, Tokyo, Mexico City

Cambridge University Press
The Edinburgh Building, Cambridge CB2 8RU, UK

Published in the United States of America by Cambridge University Press, New York

www.cambridge.org
Information on this title: www.cambridge.org/9781107683495

First published 1901
Reprinted 1924
First paperback edition 2011

A catalogue record for this publication is available from the British Library

ISBN 978-1-107-68349-5 Paperback

To Dr L. C. LANE of SAN FRANCISCO

AND TO MY OTHER MANY FRIENDS OF THAT
NEW WORLD, THE STORY OF WHOSE
LIFE IS AS YET SO SHORT BUT
MUST IN TIME BE SO GREAT,

I OFFER

AS A TOKEN OF MY FRIEND-
SHIP THIS FRAGMENT OF
THE STORY OF THE
OLD WORLD'S
LIFE

PREFACE

THE following Lectures were delivered as the "Lane Lectures" at the Cooper Medical College in San Francisco in the autumn of the past year. I have here and there expanded some parts, but otherwise the Lectures now appear very much as I delivered them. I do not pretend to have given a complete history of physiology even within the period to which I have limited myself. I have chosen certain themes which seemed to me important and striking, and I have striven to develop these, leaving untold a great deal which might be told concerning other themes. I have woven into the story of ideas, the stories of the personal lives of the men who gave birth to those ideas, partly in order to add to the human interest of the tale, but also and even more so because, in most cases at least, the fruitfulness of the labours of an inquirer is largely dependent on the inquirer's character and belongings.

I very much fear that I have allowed many mistakes in what I have written to go unnoticed and uncorrected. I may plead in excuse that historical research, perhaps above all other kinds of research, demands ample leisure, and the time which I have been able to give to the present little work has been snatched from a life broken into bits by many and varied duties. I shall be very thankful to have my mistakes pointed out.

M. FOSTER

CAMBRIDGE,
March 8, 1901

CONTENTS

LECTURE I

VESALIUS: HIS FORERUNNERS AND FOLLOWERS

I MAKE no apology for having chosen as the subject of the course of Lectures which you have honoured me by inviting me to deliver, 'The History of Physiology.' We are, all of us, even in this farthest West, even in this closing year of the nineteenth century, Children of our Fathers. What we are is in part only of our own making, the greater part of ourselves has come down to us from the past. What we know and what we think is not a new fountain gushing fresh from the barren rock of the unknown at the stroke of the rod of our own intellect, it is a stream which flows by us and through us, fed by the far-off rivulets of long ago. As what we think and say to-day will mingle with and shape the thoughts of men in the years to come, so in the opinions and views which we are proud to hold to-day, we may, by looking back, trace the influence of the thoughts of those who have gone before. Tracking out how new thoughts are linked to old ones, seeing how an error cast into the stream of knowledge leaves a streak lasting through many changes of the ways of man, noting the struggles through which a truth now rising to the surface, now seemingly lost in the depths, eventually swims triumphant on the flood we may perhaps the better learn to appraise our present knowledge, and the more rightly judge which of the thoughts of to-day is on the direct line of progress, carrying the truth of yesterday on to that of to-morrow, and which is a mere fragment of the hour, floating conspicuous on the surface now but destined soon to sink, and later to be wholly forgot.

Nor need I, I trust, make any apology for having, though invited to speak to medical hearers, chosen not the history of medicine but the history of physiology. The whole story of the rise and growth of the art of healing is too vast to be gathered into one set of lectures, too varied to be treated of by one man alone. I have chosen that part of the whole story with which alone I am competent to deal; and I venture to think that, without appearing to exalt unduly my own studies, I may go as far as to say that a knowledge of the laws which govern the phenomena of all living things is so essentially the basis of all attempts to succour, or to watch over the welfare of, one set of beings that the history of physiology cannot be regarded in any other light than as the heart or kernel of the history of medicine.

I do not propose to begin at the beginning of things. I will leave on one side, for the present at least, the details of the knowledge of the phenomena of life possessed by those whom we speak of as 'the ancients.' I will ask you to let me start with the middle of the sixteenth century, and indeed with the particular year 1543.

Those were stirring times, times of wars and rumours of wars. The brilliant career of Charles V was drawing towards its close; in that very year he was in the midst of his fourth, his last and short war with his rival Francis I of France. Venice had still all the signs of outward splendour, but within the rift in the lute was rapidly widening. The Medici were once more established at Florence, and the burly Henry VIII was ruling over England. Some twenty years before Cortez had conquered Mexico, some ten years before Pizarro had laid hold first of Peru and then of Chili; and Europe in the East was enjoying the spoils of the West.

The times were times of strong under-currents of thought. The Reformation was abroad. Luther was living his last years —he died in 1546, the year after the Council of Trent—and Calvin was strong at Geneva; but the order of the Jesuits was already a year old, and the Inquisition held Spain in its grip. It was the heyday of Art. Though Raphael had been dead for three and twenty years, Michael Angelo had nearly as many yet to live, and Titian was in his prime. The new learning was everywhere working like leaven; the old Universities were expanding and new ones were springing up everywhere, the worth of the Greek tongue was preached by the learned; and the great exponent of the oldest of sciences, that of the heavens, Nicolas Copernicus, closed his eyes in this very year. Moreover learning was being spread as well as made; printing had seen its hundredth birthday and the presses of Venice and other cities were pouring forth the means of knowledge. The night of the middle ages had passed away in the dawn of modern times.

In this year 1543 the printing-press of J. Oporinus (or Herbst) in Basel gave to the world in a folio volume the *Fabrica Humani Corporis,* the Structure of the Human Body, by Andreas Vesalius. This marked an epoch in the history of Anatomy, and so of Physiology and of Medicine. Who was Andreas Vesalius, and why did his book mark an epoch?

Let me briefly answer the latter question first. In the times of the Greeks mankind had made a fair start in the quest of natural knowledge, both of things not alive and of things living; the search had been carried on into the second century of the Christian Era when Galen expounded the structure and the use of the parts of the body of man. As Galen passed away inquiry, that is to say inquiry into natural knowledge, stood still. For a thousand years or more the great Christian Church was fulfilling its high mission by the aid of authority; but authority, as with the growth of the Church it became more and more potent as an instrument of good, became at the same time more and more potent as a steriliser of original research in natural knowledge.

The Church held the gates of learning, and they who entered were bidden to tread her path and hers alone. Her methods became the methods of all scholars. Under her guidance the written word took the place of the made world; the pursuit of truth ceased to be the looking into the phenomena of nature and the seeking for the reason why; it narrowed itself to asking what the teachers taught. The method which had proved triumphant in the search after things spiritual was taken to be the method in all inquiry, and biologic inquiry was no exception. As spiritual truths were learned by the study of the revealed word, so anatomical and medical truths were to be sought for, not by looking directly into the body of man, not by observing and thinking over the phenomena of disease, but by studying what had been revealed in the writings of Hippocrates and Galen. As the Holy Scriptures were the Bible for all men, so the works of the Greek and Latin writers became the bible for the anatomist and the doctor. Truth and science came to mean simply that which was written, and inquiry became mere interpretation.

The 'new birth' of the fifteenth and sixteenth centuries was in essence a revolt against authority as the guide in knowledge; and the work of Andreas Vesalius of which I am speaking marks an epoch, since by it the idol of authority in anatomical science was shattered to pieces never to be put together again. Vesalius described the structure of the human body such as he found it to be by actual examination, by appealing to dissection, by looking at things as they are. He dared not only to shew how often Galen was wrong, but to insist that when Galen was right he was to be followed, not because he had said it, but because what he said was in accordance with what anyone who took the pains to inquire could assure himself to be the real state of things.

Vesalius like other great men had his forerunners. Long before him at the close of the thirteenth and beginning of the fourteenth century Mundinus, Mondino (Raimondo de' Luzzi), one of the teachers of the early days of the then great University of Bologna, had dared to turn his eyes from the pages of Galen to that of nature, and to learn for himself by actual dissection how the body of man was built up. He learnt enough to write a book of his own, the *Anatomia Mundini*, which after him became a text-book in the schools, though used perhaps more as an introduction or help to Galen than in any other way. But Mundinus did not go far. He like other anatomists, like indeed Vesalius himself, had to struggle against not only the authority but the direct hand of the Church. She taught the sacredness of the human corpse, and was ready to punish as a sacrilege the use of the anatomist's scalpel; and what Mundinus did was done in the face of her powerful opposition. For this reason apparently Mundinus had no disciples carrying on his work; all that remained of him was his book, and he became little more than a smaller and a later Galen.

Two centuries later, at the very beginning of the sixteenth century, the power of the Church in its struggle against the new light was lessening, and Jacobus Berengarius, often called Carpi, from the place of his birth, a town in the state of Modena, followed in Mundinus' steps with greater éffect. He asserts that he dissected no less than a hundred corpses, and his teaching was undoubtedly to a large extent based on his own direct observations.

He too however had his struggles with the Church; he was driven to desert Bologna where he had long taught, and to live in retirement if not in exile at Ferrara. Nor did he succeed in wholly reforming anatomical science, or in placing anatomical inquiry on its only sound basis. For when he had passed away the position of Master in Anatomical Science was taken by a man of a different stamp, by Jacques Du Bois, Jacobus Sylvius, a native of Amiens, who in 1531 began to teach anatomy at Paris, and in 1550 succeeded Vidus Vidius in the Chair of Medicine at the recently established College of France.

Sylvius, though in spite of his own attitude he added to our knowledge of anatomy (we daily in the present time name him when we speak of the fissure of Sylvius), was an uncompromising Galenist. He trusted Galen more than he did his own eyes, and in everything taught or rather preached Galen. Instruction in anatomy was to him reading a chapter of Galen, and though he did make use of dissections, these were used as mere concrete illustrations to render easy the comprehension of what he was teaching, not as tests by which the truth of what he was stating might be tried.

Sylvius, as we shall see, was Vesalius' master, as indeed the master of most anatomists of the age. His influence was at the time of which we are speaking predominant; with his help the past efforts of Mundinus and of Carpi were brushed aside, and Galen and authority reigned supreme in anatomical teaching and thought. He was however the last of his school; his teaching was swept away by the new learning embodied in the *Fabrica Humani Corporis* of Andreas Vesalius.

Who then was this Andreas Vesalius?

He was born at Brussels at midnight as the last day of 1514 was passing into the first of 1515. His family, which had dwelt for several generations at Nymwegen and which originally bore the name of Witing, had produced many doctors and learned men, and his father was apothecary to Charles V. His mother, to judge by her maiden name, Isabella Crabbe, was probably of English extraction.

The young Vesalius (or Wesalius, for so it was sometimes
spelt) was sent to school at Louvain and afterwards entered
the University there, which then as later was of great renown.
Though he diligently pursued the ordinary classical and
rhetorical studies of the place, the bent of his mind early
shewed itself; while yet a boy he began to dissect such
animals as he could lay his hands on. Such a boy could not
do otherwise than study medicine, and in 1533, a lad of
seventeen or eighteen, he went to Paris to sit at the feet of
Sylvius, then rising into fame.

The ardent young Belgian was however no docile hearer,
receiving open-mouthed whatever fell from the master. Sylvius'
teaching was as I have said in the main the reading in public
of Galen. From time to time however the body of a dog or at
rarer intervals the corpse of some patient was brought into the
lecture room, and barber servants dissected in a rough, clumsy
way and exposed to the view of the student the structures
which the learned doctor, who himself disdained such menial,
loathsome work, bid them shew. This did not satisfy Vesalius.
At the third dissection at which he was present he, already
well versed in the anatomy of the dog, irritated beyond control
at the rude handling of the ignorant barbers, pushing them on
one side, completed the dissection in the way he knew it ought
to be done.

"My study of anatomy," says he, "would never have suc-
"ceeded had I when working at medicine at Paris been willing
"that the viscera should be merely shewn to me and to my
"fellow-students at one or another public dissection by wholly
"unskilled barbers, and that in the most superficial way. I
"had to put my own hand to the business."

Besides listening to Sylvius, he was a pupil of Johannes
Guinterius (Günther), a Swiss from Andernach, who also was
teaching anatomy and surgery at Paris at the time, and with
whom his relations seem to have been closer than with Sylvius.

Neither Sylvius, however, nor Guinterius, nor any one at
the time was able to supply Vesalius with that for which he
was obviously longing, the opportunity of dissecting thoroughly
the human body. Complete dissection was then well-nigh impossible, the most that could be gained was the hurried

examination of some parts of the body of a patient who had succumbed to disease. One part of the human body, the foundation of all other parts, the skeleton, could however be freely used for study. In those rude times burial was rough and incomplete, and in the cemeteries bones lay scattered about uncovered. In the burial-ground attached to the church of the Innocents at Paris Vesalius spent many hours, studying the bones; and he also tells us how in another burial-ground, on what is now 'Les Buttes Chaumont,' he and a fellow-student nearly left their own bones, being on one occasion attacked and in great risk of being devoured by savage, hungry dogs who too had come there in search of bones. By such a rough, perilous study Vesalius laid the foundation of his great work, a full and exact knowledge of the human skeleton. He tells us how he and a fellow-student were wont to try their knowledge by a test which has been often used since, the recognition of the individual bones by touch alone, with the eyes shut.

After three years the wars drove him back from Paris to Louvain, where he continued to pursue his anatomical studies with unflagging zeal. Here as at Paris he was driven to use strange means to gain the material for his studies. Walking one day with a friend in the outskirts of the city and coming to the public gibbet, where "to the great convenience of the "studious, the bodies of those condemned to death were ex- "posed to public view," they came upon a corpse "which had "proved such a sweet morsel to the birds that they had most "thoroughly cleaned it, leaving only the bones and ligaments." With his friend's help he climbed up the gallows and attempted to carry off the skeleton, but in the hurry of such a theft in open daylight he only succeeded in getting part of it; accord- ingly that evening he got himself shut out of the city gates, secured in the quiet of night the rest of the skeleton, and returning home by a roundabout way and re-entering the city by a different gate, safely carried it in.

In 1537, after a year's stay at Louvain where, in the February of that year, he put forth his first juvenile effort, a translation of the ninth book of Rhazes, he migrated to Venice, the enlightened if despotic government of which was in all possible ways fostering the arts and sciences, and striving to develop in the dependent city of Padua a University which should worthily push on the new learning. It may be worth while to note, as an instance of how in the web of man's history threads of unlike kind are made to cross, that among the monks who had charge of the Hospital at Venice, at which Vesalius pursued his medical studies, was one who bore the name of Ignatius Loyola. We may well imagine that these two young men crossed each other's path in the hospital wards or grounds, perhaps even conversed with one another. One was gathering in a rich harvest of exact knowledge which six years later he was to embody and give to the world in a great book, the beginning of modern biologic science. The other was busy with a scheme for the spiritual welfare of mankind which six years later took shape as the Order of the Jesuits. The one with his eyes fixed on man's body brought forth a work, the fruits of which have profoundly influenced and are still profoundly influencing men's minds. The other, with his eyes fixed only on truth and goodness, began that which after him became the incarnation of Authority, an engine powerful it is true for good, but often used for the support of lies and for the maintenance of evil. No two things have fought and are fighting each other more bitterly than the things which have sprung from the two works of the two young men who crossed each other's path at Venice in the year of our Lord 1537.

The brilliant talents of the young Belgian at once attracted the notice of the far-sighted rulers of Venice. He was in December of that same year, 1537, made Doctor of Medicine in their University of Padua, was immediately entrusted with the duty of conducting public dissections, and either then or very shortly afterwards, though he was but a lad of some one or two and twenty summers, was placed in a Chair of Surgery with care of Anatomy.

He at once began to teach anatomy in his own new way. Not to unskilled ignorant barbers would he entrust the task of laying bare before the students the secrets of the human frame; his own hand, and his own hand alone, was cunning enough to track out the pattern of structures which day by day were becoming more and more clear to him. Following venerated customs he began his academic labours by 'reading' Galen, as others had done before him, using his dissections to illustrate what Galen had said. But time after time the body on the table said plainly something different from that which Galen had written.

He tried to do what others had done before him, he tried to believe Galen rather than his own eyes, but his eyes were too strong for him; and in the end he cast Galen and his writings to the winds and taught only what he himself had seen and what he could make his students see too.

Thus he brought into anatomy the new spirit of the time, and the men of the time, the young men of the time answered to the new voice. Students flocked to his lectures, his hearers amounted it is said to some five hundred, and an enlightened Senate recognized his worth by repeatedly raising his emoluments.

Such a mode of teaching laid a strain on the getting of the material for teaching. Vesalius was unwearied in his search for subjects to dissect. He begged all the doctors to allow him to examine the bodies of their fatal cases. He ingratiated himself with the judges, so that when a criminal was condemned to death they gave directions that the sentence should be carried out at such a time, and the execution should be conducted now in this manner, now in that as might best meet the needs of Vesalius' public dissections. Nor did he shrink apparently from robbing the grave, for he relates how, learning of the death and hurried burial of the concubine of a monk, he got possession of the body, and proceeded at once to remove the whole of the skin in order that the peccant holy man, who had got wind of the matter, might be unable to recognize his lost love. And he made dissections in Bologna as well as Padua.

Far away from the papal throne, in distant Spain, the Church was all-powerful, and there desecration of the corpse with the knife was well-nigh impossible. In Belgium too and in France opportunities for dissection were rare. But here, in Venice, nearer the papal seat, the Church's hand was less heavy. The high-spirited citizens of the Republic were resisting as we know in many ways the Pope's demands; and under the protection of the Senate, Vesalius had opportunities for the advance of knowledge which he could not have enjoyed elsewhere.

Five years he thus spent in untiring labours at Padua. Five years he wrought, not weaving a web of fancied thought, but patiently disentangling the pattern of the texture of the human body, trusting to the words of no master, admitting nothing but that which he himself had seen; and at the end of the five years, in 1542, while he was as yet not 28 years of age, he was able to write the dedication to Charles V of a folio work, entitled the 'Structure of the Human Body,' adorned with many plates and woodcuts, which appeared at Basel in the following year, 1543. He had in 1538 published, under the sanction of the Senate of Venice, Anatomical Tables, and in the same or succeeding year had brought forth an edition of Guinterius, a treatise on blood-letting, and an edition of Galen. There is a legend that the pictures in the great work were by the hand of Titian, but there seems no doubt that they, like the Tables, were done by one John Stephen Calcar, a countryman of Vesalius.

This book is the beginning not only of modern anatomy but of modern physiology.

We cannot it is true point to any great physiological discovery as Vesalius' own special handiwork, but in a sense he was the author of discoveries which were made after him. He set before himself a great task, that of placing the study of human anatomy on a sound basis, on the basis of direct, patient, exact observation. And he accomplished it. Galen had attempted the same thing before him; but the times were not then ripe for such a step. Authority laid its heavy hand on inquiry, and Galen's teaching instead of being an example and an encouragement for further research, was, as we have said, made into a bible, and interpretation was substituted for investigation. Vesalius, inspired by the spirit of the new learning, did his work in such a way as to impress upon his age the value not only of the results at which he arrived, but also and even more so, of the method by which he had gained them. He taught in such a way that his disciples, even when they thought him greater than Galen, never made a second Galen of him; they recognized that they were most truly following his teaching as a whole when they appealed to observation to shew that in this or that particular point his teaching was wrong. After him backsliding became impossible; from the date of the issue of his work onward, anatomy pursued an unbroken, straightforward course, being made successively fuller and truer by the labours of those who came after.

Vesalius' great work is a work of anatomy, not of physiology. Though to almost every description of structure there are added observations on the use and functions of the structures described, and though at the end of the work there is a short special chapter on what we now call experimental physiology, the book is in the main a book of anatomy, the physiology is incidental, occasional, and indeed halting. Nor is the reason far to seek. Vesalius had a great and difficult task before him. He had to convince the world that the only true way to study the phenomena of the living body was, not to ask what Galen had said, but to see for oneself with one's own eyes how things really were. And not only was a sound and accurate knowledge of the facts of structure a necessary prelude to any sound conclusions concerning function, but also the former was the only safe vantage ground from which to fight against error. When he asserted that such a structure was not as Galen had described it but different, he could appeal to the direct visible proof laid bare by the scalpel. Even then he found it difficult to convince his hearers, so ready were men still to trust Galen rather than their own eyes. Much harder was the task when, in dealing with function, he had to leave the solid ground of visible fact, and to have recourse to arguments and reasoning. He seems to have said to himself, "Here am I a "young man fighting against the world; it will be enough if I "in the first instance secure a general acceptance of the truths "of structure. When I have done this, I may later on take up "the truths of function; but for the present I will not risk the "further burden which the introduction of these more debate- "able matters would entail, matters moreover about which I "clearly see that if I go very far I shall come into dangerous "conflict with the Church. I will expose, without any shrink- "ing, Galen's wrong statements about structure; but, when I "have to quote his views about function, I will expound them "without attacking them. I will content myself with letting "drop here and there a hint of my distrust and doubt."

Let me here briefly describe the main outlines of the Galenic physiology or rather of the central parts of that physiology, the features and uses of the heart and blood vessels.

The parts of the food absorbed from the alimentary canal are carried by the portal vein to the liver, and by the influence of that great organ are converted into blood. The blood thus enriched by the food is by the same great organ endued with the nutritive properties summed up in the phrase 'natural spirits.' But blood thus endowed with natural spirits is still crude blood, unfitted for the higher purposes of the blood in the body. Carried from the liver by the vena cava to the right side of the heart, some of it passes from the right ventricle through innumerable invisible pores in the septum to the left ventricle. As the heart expands it draws from the lungs through the vein-like artery (or as we now call it pulmonary vein) air into the left ventricle. And in that left cavity the blood which has come through the septum is mixed with the air thus drawn in, and by the help of that heat, which is innate in the heart, which was placed there as the source of the heat of the body by God in the beginning of life, and which remains there until death, is imbued with further qualities, is laden with 'vital spirits,' and so fitted for its higher duties. The air thus drawn into the left heart by the pulmonary vein at the same time tempers the innate heat of the heart and prevents it from becoming excessive.

Thus from the right side of the heart there is sent to the body generally along the great veins, and to the lungs along the artery-like vein (the pulmonary artery), a flow, followed by an ebb, of crude blood endued with natural spirits only, blood serving the lower stages of nutrition. Blood flows through the artery-like vein (the pulmonary artery) to the lungs for the nourishment of the lungs, just as it flows through the other veins for the nourishment of the rest of the body; in both cases there is an ebb as well as a flow along the same channel. From the left side, on the other hand, there takes place along the arteries to all parts of the body a flow, followed also by an ebb, of blood endued with vital spirits, and so capable of giving power to the several tissues to exercise their vital functions. As this blood passes from the left heart along the

vein-like artery (pulmonary vein) to the lungs it carries with
it the various fuliginous vapours which, in the fermenting
activity giving rise to the vital spirits, have been extracted
from the crude blood, and discharges these vapours into the
pulmonary passages.

Arterial blood, *i.e.* blood laden with vital spirits, reaching
the brain, there generates the animal spirits, which pure and
unmixed with blood, existing apart from blood, are carried
along the nerves to bring about movements and to carry on
the higher functions of the body.

This Galenic doctrine Vesalius was content to teach. In
his great work of 1543 he says,

"Just as the right ventricle draws blood from the cava so
"also the left ventricle draws into itself, each time the heart is
"dilated, air from the lungs through the vein-like artery, and
"uses it for the cooling of the innate heat, for the nourishment
"of its substance and for the preparation of the vital spirits,
"elaborating and refining this air so that it together with the
"blood which soaks plentifully through the septum from the
"right ventricle into the left may be assigned to the great
"artery (the aorta) and so to the whole body."

And again,

"The septum of the ventricles, composed as I have said
"of the thickest substance of the heart, abounds on both sides
"with little pits impressed in it. Of these pits, none, so far at
"least as can be perceived by the senses, penetrate through
"from the right into the left ventricle, so that we are driven to
"wonder at the handiwork of the Almighty, by means of
"which the blood sweats from the right into the left ventricle
"through passages which escape human vision."

Even in this which he ventured to print the sarcastic note
of scepticism makes itself heard; but what he really thought
he did not dare to put forward. He tells us in a later writing
that "he accommodated his statements to the dogmas of
"Galen" not because he thought that "these were in all cases
"consonant with truth but because in such a new great work
"he hesitated to lay down his own opinions, and did not dare
"to swerve a nail's breadth from the doctrines of the Prince of
"Medicine."

That physiological problems were before his mind, that he had thought over, and indeed had tried to solve them by experimental methods, is shewn in the brief chapter, 'Some Remarks on the Vivisection of Animals,' which is the last chapter in his great work. In this he relates his experiments on muscle and nerve, shewing that that which passes along a nerve in order to bring about movement passes by the substance and not by the sheath of the nerves. He tells us that it is through the spinal cord that the brain acts on the trunk and limbs, that an animal can live after its spleen has been removed, that the lungs shrink when the chest is punctured, that the voice is lost when the recurrent laryngeal nerve is cut, that by artificial respiration an animal can be kept alive though its chest is laid wholly bare, and that under these circumstances a heart which has almost stopped beating may be revived by the timely use of the bellows; and he tells us many other things.

Obviously his vigorous and active young mind was starting many inquiries of a purely physiological kind, and he was aware that much of the physiology which he had put into his book would not stand the test of future research. He knew more particularly that the chapter in that book in which he treated of the use of the heart and its parts was as he says 'full of paradoxes.' But he was no less aware that his bold attempt to expound the plain visible facts of anatomy such as they appeared to one who had torn from his eyes the bandages of authority, was of itself enough to raise a storm of opposition; he feared to jeopardize his success in that great effort by taking upon himself further burdens.

Experience shewed that in this he was right. Even while he was writing his book, timorous friends urged him not to publish it; its appearance they said would destroy his prospects in life. And in one sense it did. Towards the end of 1542 after the completion of his great task, although in August of that year he had been reappointed to the Chair of Surgery and Anatomy for three years, he, with the sanction of the Senate, left Padua for a while, his pupil Realdus Columbus being appointed his deputy. He made a short stay at Venice; he visited Basel either once or twice, chiefly it would seem to

confer with his printers; but while in that city he prepared
with his own hands from the body of an executed criminal a
complete skeleton which is still religiously preserved there. He
also probably made a hurried journey to the Netherlands.
During his absence from Padua, after the appearance of his
book the storm broke out. The great Sylvius and others
thundered against him, reviling him in a free flow of adjectives.
Coming back to Padua, after about a year's absence, he found
opposition to his new views strong even there, not the least
active among his opponents being his old pupil Columbus. He
gave lectures at Padua, offering to test publicly in the dissecting theatre whether his statements were wrong or no. He
lectured also at Bologna, and at Pisa, where the enlightened
Cosimo de' Medici of Florence would willingly have detained
him as professor in the University which he was nursing. But
such tokens of encouragement and others like them weighed
before him little when compared with the bigoted opposition
of so many of his brethren. The spirit shewn by the latter
entered like iron into his soul. If the work on which he had
laboured so long and which he felt to be so full of promise met
with such a reception, why should he continue to labour? Why
should he go on casting his pearls before swine? He had by
him manuscripts of various kinds, the embodiment of observations and thoughts not included in the *Fabrica*. What they
were we can only guess; what the world lost in their loss we
shall never know. In a fit of passion he burnt them all, and
the Emperor Charles V, offering him the post of Court
Physician, he shook from his feet in 1544 the dust of the city
in whose University he had done so much, and still a youth
who had not yet attained the thirties ended a career of science
so gloriously begun.

Ended a career; for though in the years which followed he
from time to time produced something, and in 1555 brought
out a new edition of his *Fabrica*, differing chiefly from the first
one, so far as the circulation of the blood is concerned, in its
bolder enunciation of his doubts about the Galenic doctrines
touching the heart, he made no further solid addition to the
advancement of knowledge. Henceforward his life was that
of a Court Physician much sought after and much esteemed,

a life lucrative and honourable and in many ways useful, but not a life conducive to original inquiry and thought. The change was a great and a strange one. At Padua he had lived amid dissections; not content with the public dissections in the theatre, he took parts at least of corpses to his own lodgings and continued his labours there. No wonder that he makes in his *Fabrica* some biting remarks to the effect that he who espouses science must not marry a wife, he cannot be true to both. A year after his arrival at the Court he sealed his divorce from science by marrying a wife; no more dissections at home, no more dissections indeed at all, at most some few post-mortem examinations of patients whose lives his skill had failed to save. Henceforward his days were to be spent in courtly duties, in soothing the temporary ailments, the repeated gouty attacks of his imperial master, in healing the maladies of the nobles and others round the throne, and doubtless in giving advice to more humble folk, who were from time to time allowed to seek his aid. Whither his master went, he went too, and we may well imagine that in leisure moments he entertained the Emperor and the Court with his intellectual talk, telling them some of the fairy tales of that realm of science which he had left, and of the later achievements of which news came to him, scantily, fitfully and from afar.

When in 1556 Charles withdrew from the world and took refuge in the cloister, Vesalius transferred to the son Philip II the services which he had paid to the father, and in 1559 returned with him to Spain.

Spain, as it then was, could be no home for a man of science. The hand of the Church was heavy on the land; the dagger of the Inquisition was stabbing at all mental life, and its torch was a sterilizing flame sweeping over all intellectual activity. The pursuit of natural knowledge had become a crime, and to search with the scalpel into the secrets of the body of man was accounted sacrilege. It was for a life in priest-ridden, ignorant, superstitious Madrid that Vesalius had forsaken the freedom of the Venetian Republic and the bright academic circles of Padua; in Madrid, where as he himself has said, "he "could not lay his hand on so much as a dried skull, much less "have the chance of making a dissection." Moreover, he must have felt the loss of Charles, who, whatever his faults, recognized the worth of intellectual efforts, and in many ways had shewn his sympathy with Vesalius' love of knowledge. Such sympathy could not be looked for in the narrow and bigoted Philip.

We cannot wonder that amid such surroundings the feelings that the past years had been years of a wasted life grew strong upon him, and that wistful memories of the earlier happy times gathered head. He was still in the prime of life, a man of some forty-five summers; many years of intellectual vigour were perhaps still before him. Was he to spend all these in marking time to the music of an Imperial Court?

Just at this time, in 1561, there came into his hands the anatomical observations of Falloppius (Gabrielo Falloppio), a man of whom I shall presently have to speak, who in 1551 had after a brief interval succeeded Vesalius in the Chair at Padua. This book came to the wearied and despondent Vesalius, banished to the intellectual desert of Madrid, as a living voice from a bright world outside. "Putting everything else on one "side, he gave himself," as he says, "wholly up to the instant "greedy reading of the pages" which brought vividly back to him the delights of his youth. Calling back from the past the memory of things observed long ago, for new observations, as we have seen, were out of his power, he put together bit by bit some notes criticizing Falloppius' work, put them together hurriedly and rapidly, in order that Tiepolo, the Venetian ambassador, then at Madrid but about to return to Venice, might carry the manuscript with him. In that 'Examen,' as he calls it, Vesalius says how the reading of Falloppius' notes had raised in him "a glad and joyful memory of that most "delightful life which, teaching anatomy, I passed in Italy, "the true nurse of intellects." He looks forward, he says, "to "see the ornaments of our science continue to bud forth in the "school from which I was while yet a youngster dragged away "to the dull routine of medical practice and to the worries of "continual journeys. I look forward to the accomplishment of "that great work for which, to the best of my powers so far as "my youth and my then judgment allowed, I laid foundations, "such that I need not be ashamed of them."

And even more, he was nursing the idea that his present barren life might be exchanged for a more fruitful one. "I "still," says he, "live in hope that at some time or other, by "some good fortune I may once more be able to study that "true bible, as we count it, of the human body and of the "nature of man." He was still the Vesalius of old, unchanged by all the experiences of a life at Court. The words 'that true bible' epitomize his life's works. The true bible to read is nature itself, things as they are, not the printed pages of Galen or another; science comes by observation, not by authority. And we may perhaps go so far as to suppose that by adding the words the nature of man, 'man himself,' to the words 'the body of man,' he was looking forward to doing in his riper years for physiology what in his youth he had done for anatomy.

But it was not to be. In 1563 he suddenly determined to make a pilgrimage to Jerusalem. There are various legends as to the reasons which led him to this step. It is said that in making what was supposed to be a post-mortem examination on a noble man, or according to others a woman suffering from some obscure disease, it turned out that the body was still living, and that the Church insisted upon the pilgrimage as an expiation for an act deemed to be a sacrilege. The truer account is probably that told by the botanist Clusius, that Vesalius, ill in body, and we may add even more sick at heart, wearied of the Court, and harassed by the Church, seized an opportunity, and made the proposed pilgrimage an excuse for bringing to an end his then mode of life.

On his way to Jerusalem he stopped at Venice and renewed his intercourse with scientific friends. He there learnt that the manuscript on Falloppius had never reached that anatomist, who had somewhat suddenly died in 1562, but was still in Tiepolo's hands. His friends at once obtained it from Tiepolo, and it saw the light in the following May.

The Senate at Venice were just then at a loss for a fit successor to Falloppius, and it is possible that Vesalius during his stay in the city made known his willingness to desert the Court and to return to academic life; for it is said, though documentary evidence is lacking, that during his eastern journey he received an invitation to occupy his old Chair.

Alas, on his way back in 1564 he was taken ill, or possibly a latent malady openly developed itself, he was put ashore on the island of Zante, and there he passed away.

The influence of Vesalius on the history of science may be regarded on the one hand in its general, on the other in its more special aspect.

Taking the general aspect first we may say that he founded modern anatomy. He insisted upon, and through his early unwearied labours by his conspicuous example he ensured the success of the new method of inquiry, the method of observation as against interpretation; he overthrew authority and raised up experience, he put the book of nature, the true book, in place of the book of Galen, and thus made free and open the paths of inquiry. Others before him, as we have said, Mundinus to wit and Carpi, had made like efforts, but theirs were partial and unsuccessful; Vesalius' efforts were great, complete, and successful. Upon the publication of the *Fabrica*, the pall of 'authority' was once and for ever removed. Vesalius' results were impugned, and indeed were corrected by his compeers and his followers; but they were impugned and corrected by the method which he had introduced. Inquirers asserted that in this or that point Galen was right and Vesalius was wrong, but they no longer appealed to the authority of Galen as deciding the question, they appealed now to the actual things as the judge between the two, as the judge of Galen as of others. And even those who were Vesalius' most devoted disciples never made of him a second Galen; they never appealed to him as an authority, they were content to shew on the actual body that what he had said was right.

Under a more special aspect he may be regarded as the founder of physiology as well as of anatomy in as much as he was the distinct forerunner of Harvey. For Harvey's great exposition of the circulation of the blood did, as we shall see, for physiology what Vesalius' *Fabrica* did for anatomy; it first rendered true progress possible. And Harvey's great work was the direct outcome of Vesalius' teaching, the direct outcome and yet one reached by successive steps, steps taken by men of the Italian school, of which Vesalius was the founder and father.

To these we may now turn our attention.

We have seen that even in the first edition of 1543, Vesalius hinted at his doubts about the Galenic doctrine of the uses of the heart and its parts, and that in the second edition of 1555 his doubts were more clearly outspoken. That doctrine of Galen was not merely a wrong conception of a particular part of physiology, it stood in the way of right conceptions of all parts of physiology. Let us reflect that to-day our view of any and every action and process of the body has for its fundamental basis the fact that the life of every tissue unit of the body is dependent on that unit being bathed directly or indirectly by blood which comes to it as oxygen-bearing, arterial blood, and leaves it as venous blood carrying away the products of activity. Let us remember that such a view is impossible under the Galenic doctrine which taught that to and from every tissue there was a flow and ebb of two kinds of blood, serving two purposes, one kind travelling in the veins, the other in the arteries. Let us further remember that this Galenic doctrine of the uses of veins and arteries was bound up with the Galenic doctrine of the working of the heart. If we do this we shall at once see that the true teaching of the mechanism of the bodily heart is as it were the intellectual heart of all physiology, and understand how Harvey in overthrowing the Galenic doctrine of the action of the heart, overthrew much more than that, and cleared the way for true conceptions of the actions of all parts of the body.

The central idea of the Galenic doctrine was the mysterious transit of blood from the right to the left side of the heart through the invisible pores of the septum. The transit which Galen supposed to take place was not a complete transit of the whole contents of the right ventricle, such as we now know is effected through the pulmonary circuit, but only a transit of some of the contents, the rest flowed and ebbed along the veins, just as the contents of the left ventricle flowed and ebbed along the arteries. But such a partial transit furnished the whole intercourse between the right side and the left; and all the conceptions of Galen as to what took place in the lungs, in the arteries, in the veins, and in the heart itself were dependent on the occurrence of this passage of blood through the apparently solid septum.

We have seen that it was just this part of the Galenic doctrine which excited Vesalius' strongest doubts and his most pronounced sarcasm. It was attacked also by others; some of these were Vesalius' pupils, direct or indirect, but one was not.

In Spain, in the land where above all other places the Church and the Inquisition were stifling inquiry, in Villanueva in Arragon, there was born in 1511 a man, afterwards known by the name of Michael Servetus. Fleeing early from the Inquisition and his native soil, wandering in many lands, studying many things, learning anatomy under Sylvius and Günther at Paris, where he might have sat perhaps on the same bench with Vesalius, his active mind devoured all the knowledge of the time. He was in turn jurist, astronomer, meteorologist, geographer and doctor, but above all other things, a theologian. He threw himself with zeal into medical studies, and acquired in them such a reputation that the Archbishop of Vienna made him his physician; but his real interest in such studies lay in his belief that the study of anatomy was one of the paths which lead to a knowledge of God. To know, said he, the spirit of God, we must know the spirit of man; and to truly know the spirit of man, we must know the structure and working of the body in which that spirit resides. This led him to introduce anatomical disquisitions into his theological works. These were in the main two; one was entitled *De Trinitatis Erroribus*, published in 1531, through which he stands out in history as the pioneer of Unitarian doctrine. The other, the one which most concerns us here, was the *Restitutio Christianismi*, published in 1553, but ready in manuscript long before. I need not dwell on Servetus' story here. Everyone knows how in 1553, on Oct. 27, he was burnt at the stake in Geneva at the bidding of Calvin, because he would not recant his religious faith. With him, or at the same time, there was burnt the whole edition of 1000 copies of his book, the *Restitutio*, with the exception of some few copies which had passed into the hands of friends.

In the *Restitutio* occurs this remarkable passage:

"In order, however, that we may understand how the "blood is the very life, we must first learn the generation

"in substance of the vital spirit itself which is composed and
"nourished out of the inspired air and very subtle blood. The
"vital spirit has its origin in the left ventricle of the heart,
"the lungs especially helping towards its perfection; it is a
"thin spirit, elaborated by the power of heat, of a yellow
"(light) colour, of a fiery potency so that it is as it were a
"vapour shining out of the purer blood containing the sub-
"stance of water, of air and of fire. It is generated through
"the commingling which is effected in the lungs of the
"inspired air with the elaborated subtle blood communicated
"from the right ventricle to the left. That communication
"does not, however, as is generally believed, take place through
"the median wall (septum) of the heart, but by a signal artifice
"the subtle blood is driven by a long passage through the
"lungs. It is prepared by the lungs, is rendered yellow (light)
"and from the artery-like vein is poured into the vein-like
"artery. Then in the vein-like artery it is mixed with the
"inspired air, and by expiration is cleansed from its fumes.
"And so at length it is drawn in, a complete mixture, by the
"left ventricle through the Diastole, stuff fit to become the
"vital spirit.

"That the communication and preparation does take place
"in this way through the lungs is shewn by the manifold
"conjunction and communication of the artery-like vein with
"the vein-like artery.

"This view is confirmed by the conspicuous size of the
"artery-like vein which would not have been made so large
"and so stout, and would not discharge from the heart itself
"such a power of very pure blood into the lungs for the
"mere purpose of nourishing these organs. Nor would the
"heart serve the lungs in this manner, especially since at
"an earlier date in the embryo on account of the little
"membranes of the heart, the lungs themselves are up to
"the hour of birth nourished from other sources, as Galen
"teaches."

These words shew beyond all possible doubt that Servetus
rejected wholly and unreservedly the hypothetical passage of
the blood through the septum; he went far beyond the merely
hinted scepticism of Vesalius. They further shew that he had

grasped the true features of the pulmonary circulation, the passage of the blood from the right side through the lungs to the left side. He must have attained these results by his own unaided inquiry and thought; and had he given to science the labours which he gave to theology, he obviously might have deserved the title of one of the great anatomists of the time.

But beyond the above contribution to knowledge, there is nothing in his works which can be considered as in any way marking an advance in anatomy or in physiology. Nor is there any solid reason for thinking that his writings to any extent influenced the anatomists of the time. Servetus' book, as we have seen, perished with him, only a few secret copies surviving, and there is no evidence that these survivors found their way generally into anatomists' hands; they were doubtless treasured by the theologians for whom they were written.

One point however deserves a little notice. The *Restitutio* though not published until 1553 was ready in manuscript so early at least as 1546; and there is evidence that Servetus sent manuscript copies of it in that year not only to Calvin at Geneva, but also to one Curio, a learned doctor at Padua. It has been suggested that Curio might have shewn the work, and more particularly the passage on which we have dwelt, to Vesalius, and that this is the reason why Vesalius in his edition of 1555 was more emphatic in his doubts about the passage through the septum than he had been in the first edition of 1543, before he had had the opportunity of learning Servetus' views. But this is a mere guess. Moreover even in 1543 Vesalius, as we have seen, already had his doubts, and in 1555 had he really known and accepted Servetus' statements would, we may well imagine, have spoken out with a much less uncertain sound.

I shall have something to say as to the influence Servetus' words might have had on another man, Realdo Colombo, of whom we shall have next to speak. But though it cannot be denied that Servetus was ahead of all his contemporaries in his insight into the errors of the Galenic doctrine of the heart, it is impossible to look upon him as one who exerted any marked influence on anatomical thought. He cannot be regarded as a real link in the chain which leads from Galen to Harvey and so to the present day. His utterances are of the same metal, and have the same ring as those which do form the chain, but they stand apart from these. His sayings are isolated bits of truths floating along the stream of human thought by the side of other truths, the outcome of the labours of other men.

LECTURE II

HARVEY AND THE CIRCULATION OF THE BLOOD.
THE LACTEALS AND LYMPHATICS

WHEN in 1542 after the completion of his great work Vesalius had leave to absent himself from Padua a young man Matheus Realdus Columbus, a native of Cremona, was appointed as his deputy, and when in 1544 Vesalius finally left Padua, the Senate of Venice entrusted for two years the duty of reading the lectures on Surgery and Anatomy to the same Columbus. But Columbus did not remain Vesalius' successor even for the two years; in the next year, 1545, Cosimo de' Medici appointed him as the first Professor of Anatomy in the newly renovated University of Pisa; and Vesalius' Chair was not adequately filled until 1551, when Gabrielus Falloppius was placed in it.

Falloppius, born in Modena in 1523, a favourite and a devoted pupil of Vesalius, an accomplished and travelled scholar, a careful and exact observer and describer, a faithful, modest, quiet man, has left his name in anatomy in the terms Falloppian canal and Falloppian tubes. We owe to him many valuable observations on the skeleton, especially on the skull, on the tympanum, on the muscles, and on the generative organs. But he made no large contribution to knowledge such as distinctly influenced the progress of physiology; and he left no mark on the doctrines of the circulation. I have already spoken of his Anatomical Observations as stirring up Vesalius in his later years to revived anatomical longings; in these Falloppius says that if he had been able to advance any new truth, that was largely due to Vesalius "who so shewed me "the true path of inquiry that I was able to walk along it still "farther than had been done before."

A very different man was Matheus Realdus Columbus. Born at Cremona in 1516, and therefore only a year or so younger than Vesalius, he came at the close of his 'teens' to Venice and Padua to study medicine. He says that he learnt all he knew from one Lonigo; but there can be no doubt that he also studied under and learnt much from Vesalius, who indeed says that he was very intimate with him (mihi admodum famili-aris). Apparently at first Vesalius thought very highly of his

Cremonian friend; but it was not long before the two became estranged; and with reason. Columbus was evidently a sharp, clever, man; but not only did he lack a good general education, such as Vesalius, Falloppius and others enjoyed in a high degree for they had studied Greek and philosophy as well as Latin, whereas Columbus seems to have been imperfectly acquainted even with Latin; his professional knowledge also was superficial. Vesalius spoke of him in later years as an uncultivated smatterer. So far from appreciating Vesalius' greatness, Columbus seemed to have thought that he was as good as he and that he ought to receive the like high reputation. When and wherever a Goliath appears we find some young would-be David starting up to win fame by throwing the stone at him; and Columbus, while acting as Vesalius' deputy, thought that Vesalius' absence was his opportunity, and in the anatomical theatre he insisted often and loudly on Vesalius' errors; he did his best to make Vesalius ridiculous, and to prove that the great anatomist of the time was not he but Matheus Realdus Columbus. Vesalius however on his return turned the tables on him, and thoroughly exposed his pretentions.

Again and again, in the story of the time, we find indications of something unsatisfactory about Columbus. The Venetian Archives contain two records for the year 1541, one in August nominating for the Chair of Surgery in Padua in the first place Andreas Vesalius, and in the second place Matheus Realdus Columbus, another in October confirming the above but omitting Columbus "for we wish Vesalius alone to read the "Lecture on Surgery." This suggests that the first nomination of Columbus had been gained by means of which the Senate did not approve. Later on, when in 1542 Vesalius left Padua for a while, there is evidence that Columbus, though appointed deputy, did not wholly replace the absent professor; he did the dissections, and he was probably a very skilful workman, but it would appear that one Montanus read the lecture. Lastly, upon Vesalius' final departure in 1544, though the records shew that Columbus was, as we have said, formally appointed his successor for two years certain, he only retained the Chair for a year; in 1545 he withdrew to Pisa.

The great Florentine patrons of science and art were then striving to make a famous University at Pisa. As we shall see they so far succeeded that in later years Pisa outshone Padua, Bologna and Rome; but at the time of which we are speaking, a chair at Pisa was something like a chair now-a-days in a small provincial College, a post sought after as an opportunity for winning one's spurs, a stepping-stone to better and higher things. It was such to Falloppius, who professed anatomy there from 1548 until his call to Padua in 1551. Columbus' going to Pisa was therefore not a step in the way of preferment; some other reason must have been the cause of his leaving Padua. He taught anatomy at Pisa until 1548, when he received a call to the Chair of Anatomy in the University at Rome, which he held until his early death in 1559.

He left behind him one work only, his *De Re Anatomica Libri* xv published by his children in 1559 after his death. That book though it achieved fame, and indeed Harvey spoke of its author with respect as of a great authority, is a mirror of Columbus' character and attainments. It is, though much shorter, an almost barefaced imitation of Vesalius' *Fabrica*. The frontispiece even is a bad imitation of Vesalius' frontispiece, and the work ends as does Vesalius' with a chapter on vivisection, the one being little more than a varied repetition of the other. Throughout the work are tokens of the vain man striving to exalt his own horn. He tells us again and again how much he impressed his listeners. "When I shewed "this to His Eminence, he expressed himself as hugely grati-"fied." "When I gave the demonstration of this important "new truth, I had the honour to count among my audience "His Royal Highness this, His Excellency that, and the Most "Reverend the other." He left no stone unturned with which he might hope to increase men's acknowledgment of his talents, and there are many reasons for thinking that his position at Rome was in large measure dependent on his fulsome adulation of Pope Pius IV, to whom his posthumous work was dedicated. They who know the character of Pius IV can judge of the character of the man who loaded him with praises.

Nevertheless, vain as Columbus certainly was, ignorant also in many respects as he seems to have been, there is no doubt that in the work of which we have spoken he did correctly describe the pulmonary circulation. This is what he says in his chapter on the heart and arteries:

"Two cavities, that is two ventricles, are present in the heart, "not three as Aristotle thought. Of these one is on the right "side, the other on the left. The right is much larger than "the left. The right contains the natural blood, but the left "the vital blood. It is very interesting to observe that the "substance of the heart surrounding the right ventricle is very "thin but on the left side is very thick; and this is so arranged "on the one hand in order to keep up the balance and on "the other to prevent the vital blood which is exceedingly "thin from transuding out of the heart. Between these "ventricles there is placed the septum through which almost "all authors think there is a way open from the right to the "left ventricle; and according to them the blood is in the "transit rendered thin by the generation of the vital spirits "in order that the passage may take place more easily. But "these make a great mistake; for the blood is carried by the "artery-like vein to the lung and being there made thin is "brought back thence together with air by the vein-like "artery to the left ventricle of the heart. This fact no one "has hitherto observed or recorded in writing; yet it may be "most readily observed by anyone."

And again, speaking of the vein-like artery he says:

"Anatomists, not very wise, begging their pardon, in so "doing think that the use of this is to carry the changed air to "the lungs which, like a fan, ventilate the heart, cooling this "organ and not, as Aristotle thought, the brain. The same "writers think that the lungs receive the I know not what "smoky fumes (fumos capinosos) (for so in their ignorance "of the tongues they call them) discharged from the left "ventricle. About this, all one can say is that it pleases them, "for they certainly seem to think that the same state of things "exists in the heart as in a chimney, as if there were green "logs in the heart which give out smoke when burnt. So far "concerning the use of these parts according to the opinion of "other anatomists. I for my part hold a quite different view, "namely that this vein-like artery was made to carry blood

"mixed with air from the lungs to the left ventricle of the
"heart. And this is not only most probable, but is actually
"the case; for if you examine not only dead bodies but also
"living animals, you will find this artery in all instances filled
"with blood, which by no manner of means would be the case
"if it were constructed to carry air forsooth and vapours.
"Wherefore I cannot wonder enough at those anatomists who
"have not observed a matter so clear and of such importance,
"eminent though they wish to be considered and indeed are
"considered by many of their fellows. But for these it is
"enough that Galen said so. What? To think that some
"folk in our time swear to the dogmas of Galen about anatomy
"so that they dare to assert that Galen ought to be taken as
"gospel, and that there is nothing in his writings which is not
"true! It is wonderful how men are carried away by this
"doctrine; and the princes of the anatomy offer it to the
"rabble. Yet no one sees how much this is to be blamed. Who
"indeed is there who never offends? But of this enough and
"more than enough."

He without restriction claims the discovery as his own.
Let me note in passing that he makes no attempt to draw
from the important new fact the conclusions which chiefly
give it its importance. Though he repudiates the Galenic
doctrine of the passage through the solid septum, the changed
view on this point makes no essential change in his general
views on the circulation. These still remain Galenic; the
veins still carry blood to all parts of the body. "This is the
"use of the veins, to carry blood to all parts of the body in
"order to nourish them; for all the members of the body are
"nourished by blood alone, wherefore nature made the veins
"hollow for the sake of their function that like streams they
"might pervade the body." He did not grasp the true meaning of the discovery on which he prides himself, and others
after him as we shall see also failed to see it. But did he
really himself make the discovery?

His book as we have seen was not published until 1559.
In no other writing had he published the discovery; we have
no record of when he began to teach this new doctrine of the
pulmonary circulation. He may have taught it orally to his

students, or its appearance in the posthumous work may have
been the first occasion of its being made known. We cannot
tell; but we may be well sure that he had not arrived at the
new truth before he came to Rome while he was still at Padua
or Pisa, seeking to win fame.

Now his teaching of the pulmonary circulation is almost
identical with that of Servetus, and resembles it in the absence of
the far-reaching conclusions which may be drawn from the fact.

As we have seen Servetus in 1546 sent to Curio in Padua
a manuscript copy of his *Restitutio*; this Columbus may have
seen. Again when the edition of the published *Restitutio* was
burnt in 1553, some few copies escaped; one of these may have
found its way to Rome before Columbus had sent his work
to the press.

Columbus might have taken the idea from Servetus. But
what right have we to accuse Columbus of what is in reality
a theft? Vesalius too might have seen if not Curio's manuscript
copy, at least one of the escaped prints of 1553, before he
published the second edition of his *Fabrica* in 1555. But
Vesalius does not describe the pulmonary circulation; in his
edition of 1555, he merely accentuates the doubts about the
Galenic doctrine which he felt in 1543. Columbus almost
exactly repeats Servetus' words.

Moreover we have clear evidence that in the same book
De Re Anatomica he did claim as his own discovery something
which we know he learnt from others. In that work he states
that he was the first to describe the third ossicle of the ear,
the stapes. But we know from Falloppius that the stapes
was first observed and described by John Philipp Ingrassias of
Palermo, or rather of Rachelburg, a Sicilian of eminence, who
ultimately succeeded Vesalius as physician to Philip II. Ingrassias' discovery was made known in 1548 to Falloppius, who
inquiring of his friends at Rome about it was assured by them
that neither Columbus nor any one else had ever mentioned it.

We have here evidence not only of a theft but of a bold
theft, of an unabashed attempt to assert ownership of the thing
thieved. He who sins once may be looked for to sin again; and
we may with reason suspect that Columbus' asserted discovery
of the pulmonary circulation was not his own but Servetus'.

Still the fact remains that this marked departure from the Galenic doctrine was clearly enunciated by him, and that not, as had been done by Servetus, in an out of the way manner as a link in a theological argument, but conspicuously as part of a description of the heart in an important anatomical treatise.

Of a very different stamp to Columbus was Andreas Caesalpinus. Born at Arezzo in 1519, he was for many years Professor of Medicine at Pisa, namely from 1567 to 1592, when he passed to Rome where he became Professor at the Sapienza University, and physician to Pope Clement VIII, and where at a ripe old age he died in 1603.

If Columbus lacked general culture Caesalpinus was drowned in it. Learned in all the learning of the ancients and an enthusiastic Aristotelean, he also early laid hold of all the new learning of the time. Naturalist as well as physician, he taught at Pisa Botany as well as Medicine, being from 1555 to 1575 Professor of Botany with charge of the Botanic garden founded there in 1543, the first of its kind, one remaining until the present day.

He made no marked contribution, of a clear and definite nature, to our knowledge of the structure or working of the animal body; he was indeed not an observer, but a theorist and perhaps even more a disputer. His real passion seems to have been for theology, his studies in which led him for a while into a conflict with the Church, though he ultimately recanted his heresy. His favourite doctrine was that the world was peopled with and indeed ruled by invisible demons, the apparently voluntary acts of every man being in reality the handiwork of the man's own familiar spirit. In all that related to medicine he early took up an attitude of opposition to Galen, carrying it almost to the extent of maintaining that whatever Galen affirmed was wrong, and that whatever Galen opposed was right. It would seem that it was this spirit of the controversialist rather than any careful observation of and deduction from phenomena which led him in his rambling discursive and obscurely written philosophical and medical treatises, his *Quaestiones peripateticae* (1571), and his *Questiones Medicae* (1593), to enunciate views which, however he arrived

at them, certainly foreshadowed or even anticipated those
which were later on to be established on a sound basis.

In his Peripatetic Questions he seemed to have hold of
several points relating to the true action of the heart. He
says, for instance, Lib. v. Quaest. 4:

"For the membranes are so placed at the orifices that they
"are opened when the heart is dilated and are closed when the
"heart is contracted. It follows therefore either that the lung
"and heart must be dilated at the same time and constricted at
"the same time; or the entrance of the spirits must take place
"while we breathe out. For if the heart happens to be dilated
"while the lung is constricted, and to be constricted while it is
"dilated, the air will enter the heart when we breathe out and
"issue from the heart when we breathe in; which is impossible
"for the movements are in a contrary direction. To say, how-
"ever, that the heart and lung are always dilated at the same
"time and contracted at the same time is opposed to facts,
"for we can regulate our breathing by our will, but the beat
"of the heart is wholly beyond our power; and even when we
"are breathing involuntarily, breathing is in most cases slower
"than the pulse.

"The pulse of the arteries presents another difficulty. Of
"the vessels ending in the heart, some send into it the material
"which they carry, for instance the vena cava into the right
"ventricle, and the vein-like artery into the left; some on the
"other hand carry material away from the heart, as for in-
"stance the aorta artery in the left ventricle and the artery-
"like vein nourishing the lung in the right. To each orifice are
"attached little membranes whose function is to secure that
"the orifices letting in do not lead out and that those leading
"out do not let in. It follows that when the heart contracts
"the arteries are dilated, and when it is dilated they are con-
"stricted; the two are not, it appears, constricted and dilated
"together. For when the heart is dilated, it wishes that the
"orifices of the vessels which lead out should be shut so that
"material should not flow from the heart into the arteries, but
"that it should flow in this way when the heart contracts, the
"membranes gaping (and affording a passage). If therefore
"the arteries were dilated and constricted at the same time

"as the heart, it would follow that they would be dilated at
"the time when the material filling them from the heart was
"denied them, and constricted at a time when material was
"flowing into them from it. But it is manifest that this is im-
"possible. To say therefore that the heart and arteries beat at
"different times is to deny one's senses and to doubt reason."

He thus appears to have grasped the important truth,
hidden, it would seem, from all before him, that the heart,
at its systole, discharges its contents into the aorta (and
pulmonary artery), and at its diastole receives blood from
the vena cava (and pulmonary vein).

Again, in his Medical Questions, he seems to have grasped
the facts of the flow from the arteries to the veins, and of the
flow along the veins to the heart. He says, Lib. II. Quaest. 17:

"But the following matter seems worthy of consideration,
"the reason, namely, why veins when ligatured swell on the
"far side and not on the near side of the ligature. This is a fact
"well known by experience to those who let blood; for they
"place the ligature on the near side of the place of incision,
"not on the far side, because the veins swell on the far side,
"not on the near side of the ligature. But exactly the contrary
"ought to happen if the movement of the blood and the
"spirits took place in the direction from the viscera to all parts
"of the body. When a channel is interrupted, the flow beyond
"the interruption ceases; the swelling of the veins therefore
"ought to be on the near side of the ligature.

"Here is the solution of the doubt arising from what Aris-
"totle writes concerning sleep when he says: 'It is necessary
"'that what is evaporated should be driven to some place and
"'then be turned back and changed like Euripus. For the heat
"'of every living thing ascends by nature to a higher place,
"'but when it has reached the higher place, it in many cases
"'turns back again and is carried downwards.' This is what
"Aristotle says. Now to explain this passage we must recognize
"the following. The passages of the heart are so arranged by
"nature that from the vena cava a flow takes place into the
"right ventricle, whence the way is open into the lung. From
"the lung moreover there is another entrance into the left
"ventricle of the heart, from which then a way is open into

"the aorta artery, certain membranes being so placed at the
"mouths of the vessels that they prevent return. Thus there
"is a sort of perpetual movement from the vena cava through
"the heart and lungs into the aorta artery as I have explained
"in my Peripatetic Questions.

"Now when we are awake the movement of the native heat
"takes place in a direction outwards, namely, to the sensory
"regions of the brain. When we are asleep however it takes
"place in the contrary direction towards the heart. We must
"therefore conclude that when we are awake a large supply of
"blood and of spirits is conveyed to the arteries and thence to
"the nerves. When we are asleep however the same heat is
"carried back to the heart not by the arteries but by the veins.
"For the natural entrance into the heart is furnished by the
"vena cava, not by the arteries. A proof of this may be seen in
"the pulses, which when we are wide awake are full, vehement,
"quick, with a certain rapidly repeated vibration, but when
"we are asleep are small, languid, slow and infrequent. For in
"sleep the supply of native heat to the arteries is diminished,
"but it bursts into them with vehemence when we wake. The
"veins however behave in an opposite manner; for when we
"are asleep they are more swollen, when we are awake they
"are shrunken, as anyone may see who watches the veins in
"the hands. For when we are asleep the native heat passes
"from the arteries by that communication of orifices which we
"call anastomosis into the veins and so to the heart. As how-
"ever this flowing out of blood to the higher regions, and its
"return to lower regions like a Euripus is manifest in sleep and
"wakefulness, so also a movement of the same kind is obvious
"in every part of the body to which a ligature is applied, or
"where the veins are blocked in any other way. For when its
"free channel is obstructed, a stream swells at the point
"towards which it is accustomed to flow. The blood then
"rushes forcibly back to its source, lest, being cut off, it
"should be extinguished."

We must therefore admit that Caesalpinus had not only
clearly grasped the pulmonary circulation, but had also laid
hold of the systemic circulation; he recognized that the flow
of blood to the tissues took place by the arteries and by the

arteries alone, and that the return of the blood from the tissues took place by the veins and not by the arteries.

In respect to these important points, he had obviously freed himself from the Galenic doctrine. But the question may fairly be asked, How far were these views the outcome of patient research, of real study of the phenomena themselves? How far were they flung out in the spirit of controversy as effective assaults upon accepted doctrines?

We may feel inclined to take the latter view when we notice how little acceptance Caesalpinus's new doctrines met with among his contemporaries; how little heed indeed was paid to them until they were disinterred, so to speak, by antiquarian research, and in particular what little influence they seemed to have exerted upon Caesalpinus's great contemporary who made the next great step in the advance of the true theory of the circulation, I mean Hieronymus Fabricius, often spoken of, from the place of his birth, as ab Aquapendente.

Born, in 1537, of humble parents, in the little Tuscan town or rather village bearing that name, Fabricius studied under Falloppius at Padua, and, on the death of his master, in 1565, succeeded him in the Chair of Anatomy, holding it for 40 years, until 1619, when he died at the ripe old age of 82.

A distinguished surgeon and a learned anatomist, well acquainted with the anatomy not only of man but of other vertebrates, he was the author of many treatises, most of which had distinct physiological bearings and which contained many contributions to the advancement of knowledge. He was the first after Aristotle to describe the formation of the chick in the egg; he wrote well on locomotion, on the eye, on the ear, on the skin, on the larynx and on speech; but the one work which concerns the subject which we have in hand is that on the valves of the veins, the book *De venarum ostiolis*, 'the little doors of the veins,' which saw the light in 1574.

Johannus Baptista Cannanus, Professor at Ferrara, is said to have observed the valves long before, namely in 1547, and indeed to have told Vesalius of his observation; and even before that, these structures it is said were noticed by Sylvius. But they were not really laid hold of until Fabricius published his book. In that work he most carefully and accurately

described their structure, position and distribution, illustrating his observations by fairly good figures. He moreover
clearly recognized that the valves offered opposition to the
flow of blood from the heart towards the periphery, and even
gives the now well-known demonstration of their action on
the living arm.

He says, *De venarum ostiolis*:

"Little doors of the veins is the name I give to certain very
"thin little membranes occurring on the inside of the veins,
"and distributed at intervals over the limbs, placed sometimes
"one by itself, and sometimes two together. They have their
"mouths directed towards the root of the veins (*i.e.* the heart),
"and in the other direction are closed. Viewed from the outside
"they present an appearance not unlike the swellings which
"are seen in the branches and stem of a plant. In my opinion
"they are formed by nature in order that they may to a
"certain extent delay the blood and so prevent the whole of it
"flowing at once like a flood either to the feet, or to the hands
"and fingers, and becoming collected there. For this would
"give rise to two evils; on the one hand the upper parts of the
"limbs would suffer from want of nourishment, and on the
"other the hands and feet would be troubled with a continual
"swelling. In order therefore that the blood should be every-
"where distributed in a certain just measure and admirable
"proportion for maintaining the nourishment of the several
"parts, these valves of the veins were formed.

*   *   *   *   *   *   *

"In the veins laid bare and examined untouched, these
"valves are visible to a certain extent. Nay more, that even
"in the living arm or thigh these valves may give evidence of
"their existence appears clearly from the fact that, when in
"letting blood the assistants bind the limbs, at intervals along
"the course of the veins, little knots as it were are seen from
"the outside; these are swellings caused by the valves.

*   *   *   *   *   *   *

"That indeed the flow of the blood is slowed by means
"of these valves is not only made clear by their construction
"but also is shewn by the following experiment which anyone

"can make, either by laying bare the veins in a dead body, or "by ligaturing a limb in a living body, as they do when they "let blood. For if you attempt to press, or by rubbing to drive "the blood downwards (towards the hand for instance) you "will clearly see that its flow is prevented and delayed by the "valves."

But he wholly failed to recognize their true function. Still labouring under the influence of the old doctrines and believing that the use of the veins was that of carrying crude blood, blood not vivified by the vital spirits, from the heart to the tissues, he thought that he had fully explained the value of the veins, by pointing out that they opposed the flow from the heart to the tissues, not of all blood but only of an excess of blood; their purpose was to prevent the blood as it flowed along the veins from the heart being heaped up too much in one place. But he also thought that they were the means of furnishing temporary local reservoirs of blood; and he likens them to the devices by which in mills and elsewhere water is dammed up. He left for another, for a pupil of his, the opportunity of putting to its right use the discovery which he had made.

Though he wrote on many points of physiology, Fabricius did not grapple with the problems of the heart. We learn his views on these incidentally from his treatise, *De respiratione et ejus instrumentis*, written in 1599, but not published until 1603. The greater part of this work deals and deals well with the muscles and with the general mechanism of respiration, but in it he also speaks of the relation of respiration to the work of the heart.

In view of the importance of rightly appreciating the value of the great work which was to appear a quarter of a century later, it may be worth while to ask what were the views concerning the circulation which at the close of the sixteenth century were being expounded by this great teacher, whose lectures were attended by such crowded classes, that a new great theatre had to be built for him, who was drawing hearers to him, not only from all Italy, but from all parts of Europe, even from distant Britain, and who by his fame maintained and even increased the reputation of the great school of Padua.

Strange as it may seem, the teaching of Fabricius in 1599 was little more than a repetition of the teaching of Galen; and it is worthy of notice that in this treatise, while he repeatedly refers to Galen, he hardly at all refers to Vesalius, or to any other modern anatomist.

This is what he says:

"Admitting then that the lungs are composed of their own "proper tissue, of the artery-like vein, of the vein-like artery "and of the rough artery (trachea), and that they possess the "artery-like vein for the purposes of their own nourishment, "that they possess their own proper tissue to act like tow for "the purpose of supporting and guarding the terminations of "the vessels, and that they possess the rough artery, in order "that there may be a fit receptacle for receiving the air, "admitting this, it would nevertheless seem altogether reason-"able to think that the whole construction of the lungs was "carried out chiefly for the sake of the remaining vessel, "namely, the vein-like artery which seizes upon the air in "the lungs and carries it to the heart, the same forsooth being "drawn through them by the heart. It is thus reasonable to "suppose that the lungs exist for the sake of the vein-like "artery, the use of which is that the air may conveniently "reach the heart; for otherwise the air would be drawn into "the cavity of the thorax and would never reach the heart "did not the heart extend its vein-like artery from its left "sinus right up into the lungs."

And in his Epilogus he thus sums up:

"In breathing, Nature puts before herself mainly a double "goal, the generation of the animal spirits, and the regulation "and conservation of the heat of the heart. The heat is main-"tained and regulated by the supply of material, by refrigera-"tion, and by getting rid of superfluous residues. All these "things are brought about by means of the air taken into the "body, whence the necessity of breathing. This breathing is "the bringing in of air by which spirit is carried inwards and "outwards through the mouth, and is divided into inspiration "and expiration. In inspiration air enters the lungs and the "heart for the sake of the supply of material and of refrigera-"tion; in expiration, on the other hand, the air issues for the

"sake of getting rid of superfluous residues. The air enters by
"being drawn in, it issues by being driven out; it is drawn
"in, not by any occult virtues or influences, but only by the
"principle that a vacuum must be filled up."

In spite of many clear views as to the mechanics of respiration, he holds that the air is carried to the heart by the
vein-like artery, and much of his work is taken up in a long
discussion as to the exact way in which the air thus entering
affects on the one hand the generation of the vital spirits, and
on the other hand the innate heat of the heart.

"If all this belongs to the innate heat of the heart which
"burns as with a flame, it must in any case be maintained that
"the whole business of maintaining and regulating that heat
"consists in the first place of providing material (for the flame),
"then of ventilation, then of moderate refrigeration, and lastly
"of the discharge of fumes; all these are supplied by respira-
"tion."

In his treatise on the formation of the fœtus he says:

"The lungs while (in the adult) they are doing work for the
"good of the whole body, make use in the following manner of
"the three kinds of vessels which penetrate their substance,
"namely, the rough artery, the artery-like vein, and the vein-
"like artery. By means of the rough artery they are the first
"to seize upon and receive the air drawn in by respiration,
"which subsequently by the beat of the heart is carried
"through the vein-like artery into the left cavity of the heart,
"to be elaborated and converted into vital spirits and at the
"same time to afford refrigeration for the heart. By means of
"the third vessel, which is spoken of as the artery-like vein,
"the lungs are nourished with the purest and thinnest blood.
"Hence, during this time, the lung is nourished by a vessel
"possessing the structure of an artery, but indeed receives
"spirits by a vessel which has the substance of a vein. But
"while the fœtus is being carried in the uterus, since the lung
"does not carry out the function of respiration, but attends
"only to its own business, the change of function is accom-
"panied by a change of structure. For it lays hold of blood
"for its own nutrition by means of the venous vessel, but
"draws in vital spirits by an arterial vessel."

All this is sheer Galenism, with here and there a modern touch. It may be worth while to call to mind that the man who in 1599 wrote this was the pupil, a favourite pupil, of Falloppius, who was in turn the favourite pupil of Vesalius, and that the atmosphere around the Chair of Anatomy at Padua must have been thick with the memories and traditions of the teachings of these great men.

He had probably heard Falloppius tell many a saying of Vesalius, many an expression of the great man's not embodied in the written work. He probably bade his hearers take Vesalius' great work as their text-book, that great work in which Vesalius, by his insistence of the value of original inquiry as against the mere following of authority, and no less by the free expression of his doubts concerning current doctrines and of the need of putting these to the test of examination, had boldly cleared the way for future research. Even if he had not read Servetus, he must have been familiar with Columbus's book; and both of these (we may lay on one side for the moment the possible connection between the two) had declared against the mysterious passage through the solid septum and in favour of the flow through the lungs, from the right side to the left side of the heart. He could not have been ignorant of the writings of Caesalpinus, who had so boldly expounded his views as to the action of the heart, and the flow along the veins from the tissues to the heart. He himself had contributed that knowledge of the valves of the veins, which rightly used overturned the whole Galenic doctrine. Yet it was then, as it is now to-day, as it has been in every period between then and now, as it was in all times before, and as it will be so far as we can see in all times to come. So strong was the hold upon his mind of conceptions coming down from the past, that Fabricius's eyes were blinded to facts staring him in the face, and his ears were deaf to voices crying out new views. At almost the very parting of the ways he continued calmly to preach that the old way was the better one, the way in which men should walk.

It was left for a pupil of his to seize that which he had just failed to lay hold of, to weld together, as he was passing away, into one sustained and convincing argument, the several links which he and the rest had furnished, and nine years after his death to make known to the world that true view of the circulation which was the real beginning of modern physiology.

I need not take up time by entering largely into the details of the oft-told story of William Harvey's life.

Born at Folkestone, on the south coast of England, in April 1578, just four years after Fabricius had published his treatise on the valves of the veins, admitted to Gonville and Caius College, Cambridge, in 1593, taking his degree in Arts in 1597, he left England the following year to study medicine under the great master at Padua. There he spent the greater part of four years, years very nearly overlapping the period between the writing and the publication of Fabricius's treatise on Respiration, of which I have just spoken as being, in great measure, an exposition of the Galenic doctrine of the circulation. At the end of the period, in 1602, he received at Padua the degree of Doctor of Medicine, and on his return to England in the same year was incorporated into the Doctorate at Cambridge.

Setting up his abode in London, joining the Royal College of Physicians in 1604, and becoming Physician to St Bartholomew's Hospital in 1609, he ventured in 1615 to develop, in his Lectures on Anatomy at the College of Physicians, the view which he was forming concerning the movements of the heart and of the blood. But his book, his *Exercitatio*, on that subject did not see the light until 1628.

'The little choleric man,' as Aubrey calls him, attained fame among his fellows, and favour at Court. As Physician to King Charles I he accompanied that monarch on his unhappy wanderings, and every one knows the tale or legend of how at the battle of Edgehill, taking care of the Princes he sat, on the outskirts of the fight under a hedge, reading a book. In 1646, after the events at Oxford, he retired into private life, publishing in 1651 his treatise, *De generatione animalium*, in which he followed up some of the researches of his Paduan master, and on June 3, 1667, he ended a life remarkable for its effects rather than for its events.

It is a fashion to speak of Harvey as 'the immortal Discoverer of the Circulation'; but the real character of his work is put in a truer light when we say that he was the first to demonstrate the circulation of the blood. His wonderful book, or rather tract, for it is little more, is one sustained and condensed argument, but an argument founded not on general principles and analogies but on the results of repeated 'frequent appeals to vivisection' and ocular inspection. He makes good one position, and having done that advances on to another, and so marches victoriously from position to position until the whole truth is put clearly before the reader, and all that remains is to drive the truth home by further striking illustrations.

His first position is the true nature and purpose of the movements of the heart itself, that is of the ventricles. When, in the beginning of the inquiry, he 'first gave his mind to vivisections' he found the task of understanding the 'motions and uses of the heart so truly arduous, so full of difficulties' that he began to think with Fracastorius (a Veronese doctor of the middle of the sixteenth century (1530) and more a poet than a man of science), "that the motion of the heart was only "to be comprehended by God." But the patient and prolonged study of many hearts of many animals shewed him that "the "motion of the heart consists in a certain universal tension, "both of contraction in the line of its fibres, and constriction in "every sense, that when the heart contracts it is emptied, that "the motion which is in general regarded as the diastole of the "heart is in truth its systole," that the active phase of the heart is not that which sucks blood in, but that which drives blood out. Caesalpinus alone, as we have seen, of all Harvey's forerunners had in some way or other dimly seen this truth. Harvey saw it clearly and saw it in all its consequences. It is, he says, the pressure of the constriction, of the systole, which squeezes the blood into and along the arteries, it is this transmitted pressure which causes the pulses; the artery swells at this point or that along its course, not in order that it may suck blood into it, but because blood is driven into it, and that by the pressure of the constricting systole of the heart.

With this new light shining in upon him, he was led to a clear conception of the work of the auricles and the ventricles, with their respective valves. He saw how the vena cava, on the one side, and the vein-like artery, the pulmonary veins, on the other side, empty themselves into and fill the ventricles during the diastole, and how the ventricles in turn empty themselves during the systole into the artery-like vein, the pulmonary artery on the one side and the great artery or aorta on the other. And this at once led him to a truer conception of the pulmonary circulation than was ever grasped by Servetus or Columbus. On the old view, only *some* of the blood of the right ventricle passed through the septum into the left ventricle; the rest went back again to the tissues; and it was this 'some' only which Servetus and Columbus believed to pass through not the septum but the lungs. Harvey saw that all the reasons for thinking that any of the contents of the ventricle so passed were equally valid for thinking that all passed, and that the latter view alone was consonant with the facts.

This new view, new in reality, though having so much resemblance to old ones that Harvey speaks of it as one "to "which some, moved either by the authority of Galen or "Columbus or the reasonings of others, will give their ad- "hesion," led him at once to another conception which how- ever "was so new, was of so novel and unheard of a character "that in putting it forward he not only feared injury to him- "self from the envy of a few, but trembled lest he might have "mankind at large for his enemies." This new view consisted simply in applying to the greater circulation the same con- clusions as those at which he had arrived in regard to the lesser circulation.

It is important to note that to this new view he was guided by distinctly quantitative considerations. He argued in this way. At each beat of the heart a quantity of blood is trans- ferred from the vena cava to the aorta. Even if we take a low estimate (he had made observations with a view to deter- mining the exact amount but he leaves this aside for the present as unessential), say half an ounce, or three drachms, or only one drachm, and multiply this by the number of beats, say in half-an-hour, we shall find that the heart sends through the arteries to the tissues during that period as much blood as is contained in the whole body. It is obvious, therefore, that the blood which the heart sends along the arteries to the tissues cannot be supplied merely by that blood which exists in the veins as the result of the ingesta of food and drink; only a small part can be so accounted for; the greater part of that blood must be blood which has returned from the tissues to the veins; the blood in the tissues passes from the arteries to the veins, in some such way as in the lungs it passes from the veins (through the heart) to the arteries; the blood moves in a circle from the left side of the heart, through the arteries, the tissues and the veins to the right side of the heart, and from thence through the lungs to the left side of the heart.

This is what he says:

"I frequently and seriously bethought me, and long revolved "in my mind, what might be the quantity of blood which was "transmitted, in how short a time its passage might be effected, "and the like; and not finding it possible that this could be "supplied by the juices of the ingested aliment without the "veins on the one hand becoming drained, and the arteries on "the other hand becoming ruptured through the excessive "charge of blood, unless the blood should somehow find its way "from the arteries into the veins, and so return to the right "side of the heart; I began to think whether there might not "be *a motion, as it were, in a circle*. Now this I afterwards "found to be true; and I finally saw that the blood, forced by "the action of the left ventricle into the arteries, was dis- "tributed to the body at large, and its several parts, in the "same manner as it is sent through the lungs, impelled by the "right ventricle into the pulmonary artery, and that it then "passed through the veins and along the vena cava, and so "round to the left ventricle in the manner already indicated, "which motion we may be allowed to call circular."

As the sun of this truly new idea rose in Harvey's mind, this new idea that the blood is thus for ever moving in a circle, the mists and clouds of many of the conceptions of old faded away and the features of the physiological landscape hitherto hidden came into view sharp and clear. This idea once grasped, fact after fact came forward to support and enforce it. It was now clear why the heart was emptied when the vena cava was tied, why it was filled to distension when the aorta was tied. It was now clear why a middling ligature which pressed only or chiefly on the veins made a limb swell turgid with blood, whereas a tight ligature which blocked the arteries made it bloodless and pale. It was now clear why the whole or nearly the whole of the blood of the body could be drained away by an opening made in a single vein. And now for the first time was clear the purpose of those valves in the veins, whose structure and position had been demonstrated doubtless to Harvey, by the very hands of their discoverer, his old master Fabricius, but "who did not rightly understand their use, and "concerning which succeeding anatomists have not added "anything to our knowledge."

Fabricius, as we have seen, had used the now well-worn experiment of pressing on the cutaneous veins of the bared arm to demonstrate the existence of the valves; but he had used it to demonstrate their existence only. Blinded by the conceptions of his time he could not see that the same experiment gave the lie to his explanation of the purpose of the valves, and demonstrated not only their existence, but also their real use. Harvey, with the light of his new idea, at once grasped the true meaning of the knotty bulgings.

These however were not the only phenomena which now for the first time received a reasonable explanation. Harvey was able to point to many other things; to various details of the structure and working of the heart, to various phenomena of the body at large both in health and in disease as intelligible on his new view, but incomprehensible on any other.

If we trust, as indeed we must do, Harvey's own account of the growth of this new idea in his own mind, we find that he was not led to it in a straight and direct way by Fabricius' discovery of the valves. It was not that the true action of these led to the true view of the motion of the blood, but that the true view of the motion of the blood led to the true understanding of their use. To that true view of the motion of blood he was led by a series of steps, each in turn based on observations made on the heart as seen in the living animal, or as he himself says 'repeated vivisections,' the great step of all being that one by which he satisfied himself that the quantity of blood driven out from the heart could not be supplied in any other way than by a return of the blood from the arterial endings in the body through the veins. As he himself says: "Since all things, both argument and ocular demonstration, "shew that the blood passes through the lungs and heart by "the action of the ventricles, and is sent for distribution to all "parts of the body, where it makes its way into the veins and "pores of the flesh, and flows by the veins from the circum- "ference on every side to the centre, from the lesser to the "greater veins, and is by them finally discharged into the vena "cava and right auricle of the heart, and this in such a quan- "tity or in such a flux and reflux thither by the arteries, hither "by the veins, as cannot possibly be supplied by the ingesta, "and is much greater than can be required for mere purposes "of nutrition; it is absolutely necessary to conclude that the "blood in the animal's body is impelled in a circle, and is in "a state of ceaseless motion; that this is the act or function "which the heart performs by means of its pulse; and that it "is the sole and only end of the motion and contraction of the "heart."

Harvey's argument is essentially a physical mechanical argument; the problem which he puts before himself to solve is essentially a mechanical physical problem; the solution of that problem at which he arrived is essentially a mechanical solution of the phenomena of the circulation. As we have seen, in the minds of those before him the mechanical problems of the circulation were mixed up with questions about the dis- tribution of the various kinds of spirits, the natural, vital and animal spirits. With these questions Harvey does not deal at all. In an early passage he says, "Whether or not the heart, "besides propelling the blood giving it motion locally and "distributing it to the body, adds anything else to it—heat, "spirit, perfection—must be inquired into by and by, and "decided upon other grounds." And never again, throughout the whole of his argument, does he refer to the questions of the spirits.

Yet his demonstration was the death-blow to the doctrine of the 'spirits.' The names it is true survived for long after- wards, but the names were henceforward devoid of any really essential meaning. For the view of the natural and vital spirits was based on the supposed double supply of blood to all the tissues of the body, the supply by the veins carrying natural spirits and the supply by the arteries carrying vital spirits. The essential feature of Harvey's new view was that the blood through the body was the same blood, coursing again and again through the body, passing from arteries to veins in the tissues, and from veins to arteries through the lungs, heart, suffering changes in the substance and pores of the tissues, changes in the substance and pores of the lungs.

The new theory of the circulation made for the first time possible true conceptions of the nutrition of the body, it cleared the way for the chemical appreciation of the uses of blood, it afforded a basis which had not existed before for an understanding of how the life of any part, its continued existence and its power to do what it has to do in the body, is carried on by the help of the blood. And in this perhaps, more than its being a true explanation of the special problem of the heart and the blood vessels, lies its vast importance.

We shall see presently how the new way thus opened up by Harvey was followed with brilliant success, on the one hand in England, and on the other hand in Italy. Meanwhile it may be well to turn aside to tell in a brief way the story of a special but yet important addition to our knowledge of the blood system, which was being made at the very time that Harvey was meditating over and developing his views.

That the food which disappears from the alimentary canal, during its passage along it, becomes in some way or other blood, was a view which took origin in the early days of mankind so soon as man began to consider what took place within his frame. It was part of the Galenic doctrine that the food thus utilized for the body was taken up from the alimentary canal by the vena porta and carried to the liver, there to be enriched with the natural spirits and so concocted into the blood which passed on to the heart.

Galen himself quotes Erasistratus as having seen that, in young kids which had lately sucked, the arteries in the mesentery contained milk, and indeed had observed the same thing himself. Eustachius too, the anatomist of Rome, who flourished between Vesalius and Fabricius, whose name and labours are preserved among us by the Eustachian tube and Eustachian valve, saw apparently what we now call the thoracic duct. Nevertheless it may be said that up to the early years of the seventeenth century, anatomists were aware of one set of vessels only, the blood vessels, arterial or venous.

In the year 1622 Gaspar Aselli of Cremona, Professor of Anatomy at Pavia, discovered the lacteals; and this is how he relates his discovery:

"On the 23rd of July of that year (1622) I had taken a "dog in good condition and well fed, for a vivisection at the "request of some of my friends, who very much wished to see "the recurrent nerves. When I had finished this demonstra- "tion of the nerves, it seemed good to watch the movements "of the diaphragm in the same dog, at the same operation. "While I was attempting this, and for that purpose had "opened the abdomen and was pulling down with my hand "the intestines and stomach gathered together into a mass, "I suddenly beheld a great number of cords as it were, "exceedingly thin and beautifully white, scattered over the "whole of the mesentery and the intestine, and starting from "almost innumerable beginnings. At first I did not delay, "thinking them to be nerves. But presently I saw that I was "mistaken in this since I noticed that the nerves belonging to "the intestine were distinct from these cords, and wholly "unlike them, and, besides, were distributed quite separately "from them. Wherefore struck by the novelty of the thing, "I stood for some time silent while there came into my mind "the various disputes, rich in personal quarrels no less than "in words, taking place among anatomists concerning the "mesaraic veins and their function. And by chance it happened "that a few days before I had looked into a little book by "Johannes Costaeus written about this very matter. When I "gathered my wits together for the sake of the experiment, "having laid hold of a very sharp scalpel, I pricked one of "those cords and indeed one of the largest of them. I had "hardly touched it, when I saw a white liquid like milk or "cream forthwith gush out. Seeing this, I could hardly "restrain my delight, and turning to those who were standing

"by, to Alexander Tadinus, and more particularly to Senator
"Septalius, who was both a member of the great College of the
"Order of Physicians and, while I am writing this, the Medical
"Officer of Health, 'Eureka' I exclaimed with Archimedes,
"and at the same time invited them to the interesting
"spectacle of such an unusual phenomenon. And they indeed
"were much struck with the novelty of the thing."

Aselli detected the presence of valves in these vessels and
recognized that they hindered the backward flow. He saw
clearly indeed that his newly discovered vessels were channels
for conveying the chyle, the elaborated contents of the intestine, away from the intestine; but influenced doubtless by
the accepted view that all the absorbed food must be carried
to the liver to be there elaborated into blood, he went wrong
as to the ultimate course taken by these vessels; he could trace
them he thought into the liver. It may here be noted in
passing that Aselli in his treatise speaks of and indeed figures
the cluster of lymphatic glands lying in the mesentery as 'the
pancreas'; and this cluster of glands was afterwards often
spoken of as 'the pancreas of Aselli.'

Aselli's discovery by itself was not perhaps of capital
importance; and indeed for a quarter of a century it remained
an isolated and barren bit of knowledge. After that interval,
however, Jean Pecquet, a French physician who practised first
in Dieppe and subsequently in Paris, in his *Experimenta nova
anatomica*, published in Paris in 1651, made known a further
discovery, one which he says he had come upon years before
while studying at Montpellier, the discovery of the receptacle
of the chyle and its continuation as the thoracic duct. Pecquet
not only accurately describes these structures, but shews that
on the one hand Aselli's lacteals pour their contents into the
receptacle, and that on the other the thoracic duct, the continuation of the receptacle, pours its contents into the venous
system at the junction of the jugular and subclavian veins.
In the following year, 1652, Van Horn made known the same
discovery, which he appears to have arrived at quite independently of Pecquet.

By this discovery of the thoracic duct and its entrance into
the veins, a wholly new aspect was given to Aselli's original

observation. The mere existence of special vessels such as the lacteals in the mesentery was quite consistent with, indeed supported, the old views of the circulation. Pecquet's observation was wholly inconsistent with them; but between Aselli and Pecquet, Harvey's book had appeared; and it may be taken as a proof of how profoundly Harvey's arguments had in so short a time influenced men's minds, that Pecquet's observations, which if put forward thirty years before would have been rejected as impossible, were now accepted without misgivings. Indeed they afforded no little support to the new theory of the circulation.

Further support was supplied almost at the same time by the publication in 1653 of the *Nova exercitatio anatomica* of Olaus Rudbeck, Professor of Anatomy and also of Botany in the University of Upsala (after whom is named the genus Rudbeckia). In this treatise Rudbeck described under the name of *vasa serosa* or *aquosa*, or *ductus serosi*, *aquosi*, vessels like the lacteals in structure, but containing not milk, or chyle, but a clear watery liquid, vessels which we now call lymphatics. He saw them first in the liver and intestines and traced them to the thoracic duct, of whose existence, he says, he became aware in 1650 before the publication of Pecquet's book. We learn from Glisson that one Jolive, an Englishman, in taking his Doctor's degree at Cambridge in 1652, presented in his thesis an account of these same lymphatics, and by some authors priority in the matter is thereby claimed for him.

Within a few years then of the publication of Harvey's book, anatomists became aware of a new set of vessels, of whose existence no one before had dreamed, vessels neither arteries nor veins, vessels containing not blood but either a milky or a clear limpid fluid, and carrying their contents not to but away from the tissues, carrying them moreover not to that great organ the liver, which in the old view was the chief seat of all concoction, but directly into the venous blood stream and so to the heart, from thence to be distributed all over the body. That such a conception almost at once found general acceptance is, as we have just said, a striking proof of how rapidly and profoundly Harvey's work had influenced the views of physiologists.

When Aselli first discovered his lacteals he very naturally concluded that all the chyle, the whole of the nutritive and absorbable contents of the alimentary canal, found its way into the system through them. It is interesting to note that Harvey hesitated to accept this conclusion. In a letter to Morison at Paris written in April 1652, a year after the publication of Pecquet's treatise, he says:

"With regard to the lacteal veins discovered by Aselli, and "by the further diligence of Pecquet, who discovered the "receptacle or reservoir of the chyle, and traced the canals "thence to the subclavian veins, I shall tell you freely, since "you ask me, what I think of them. I had already in the "course of my dissections, I venture to say even before Aselli "had published his book, observed these white canals,......But "for various reasons, and led by several experiments, I could "never be brought to believe that that milky fluid was chyle "conducted hither from the intestines, and distributed to all "parts of the body for their nourishment; but that it was "rather met with occasionally and by accident, and proceeded "from too ample a supply of nourishment and a peculiar "vigour of concoction."

And he goes on to argue against the probability of all the material solid and liquid absorbed from the alimentary canal taking this path of the lacteals only. "Why indeed should we "not as well believe that the chyle (digested contents of the "intestine) enters the mouth of the mesenteric veins and in "this way becomes immediately mingled with the blood where "it might receive digestion and perfection......And that the "thing is so in fact, I find an argument in the distribution of "innumerable arteries and veins to the intestines, more than "to any other part of the body, in the same way as the uterus "abounds with blood vessels during the period of pregnancy."

With Harvey's demonstration of the circulation of the blood, supplemented as it was with the discovery of the lymphatics, physiology was almost suddenly transformed. Harvey's work had a double effect. In the first place it rendered possible an exact inquiry into the properties and functions of the organs and tissues of the body. So long as the blood in the arteries and in the veins were looked upon as two different kinds of waves as it were, breaking upon and ebbing from the tissues, the one carrying vital, and the other natural spirits, there seemed to be no opening for any attempts to explain the phenomena exhibited by this or that part, this or that organ or tissue on physical or mechanical principles; everything was wrapped up in the mystery of the spirits. So soon however as it was recognized that the blood which was carried to a part along the arteries came back away from the part along the veins, the same blood, altered it might be in the transit but still the same blood, such attempts became at once possible. The spirits became at once mere qualities of the blood, their names might be retained, but the virtue had gone out of the names; the names were no longer a hindrance to exact inquiry as to what took place in an organ when it entered into a phase of activity and how that activity was influenced by or influenced the blood.

In the second place Harvey's work was a shining example for all future inquirers. The patient examination of anatomical features, if possible a comparison of those features in the same organ or part in more animals than one, the laying hold of some explanation of the purpose of those features suggested by the features themselves, and the devising of experiments, by vivisection or otherwise, which should test the validity of that explanation, that was Harvey's threefold method. It had it is true been followed before, by Vesalius and succeeding anatomists, and indeed in a measure by Galen himself; but these had for the most part been content with the explanation suggested by structure, and had rarely used the test of experiment, though as we have seen Vesalius at least saw its value. It was Harvey's great merit to have boldly used the experimental method, to have set a lesson, to the zealous following of which the progress of physiology after him has been largely due.

All great men have their detractors; and Harvey has been no exception. Many writers have attempted to claim for others than him the credit of his great work. To Servetus, Realdus Columbus and Caesalpinus and to others has been attributed in turn the merit of the discovery of circulation. I trust I have been able to put in a clear light what were the several contributions to the progress of knowledge of the above three men, and how wholly they fell short of Harvey. I need not tarry to speak of Carlo Ruini of Bologna, who, though no professor, wrote in 1598 a very admirable book on the Anatomy of the Horse, in which he shewed that he had grasped, in a striking manner, the actions of the valves of the heart. One name however needs to be dealt with, that of Petrus Paulus Sarpi, the brilliant Venetian, theologian, philosopher, and martyr. Sarpi studied anatomy as indeed he studied all the sciences of his time, and he studied it under Fabricius. Now, one Thomas Cornelius Consentinus is the author of the story that Sarpi, while he was studying at Padua, arrived at conclusions concerning the circulation of the blood identical with those of Harvey, conclusions developed in a manuscript found among his papers after his death. The story goes on to say that Sarpi had made known his conclusions to his master Fabricius, who did not himself think much of them, but told his pupil Harvey about them; and Harvey going home to England published them as his own.

But Ent in his *Apologia* gives a very different version. He says that the Venetian Legate returning from London to Venice carried with him a copy of Harvey's book, which had just appeared. This copy he lent to Sarpi, and the latter was so struck with the new views that he transcribed for his own use very much of the lent book. It was this transcription of Harvey which Sarpi's heirs found among his papers after his death.

All such attempts to take away from Harvey what is his due are vain and useless efforts. The greatness of all great men is partly built on the worth of those who have gone before. In science no man's results are wholly his own, like other living things they come from something which lived before. Vesalius, Servetus, Fabricius and the rest led up to Harvey; but they were not Harvey. He was himself, and his greatness is in no wise lessened by its having come through them.

LECTURE III

BORELLI AND THE INFLUENCE OF
THE NEW PHYSICS

HARVEY'S method of inquiry was that which may be called
the purely or strictly physiological method. Observing carefully the phenomena of the living body, he sought in the first
place, in the arrangements of the structures concerned in the
facts of anatomy, for suggestions as to how the phenomena
might be explained. It is this aspect of his method which
brings into striking light the value of the work of Vesalius and
of the school of Vesalius as the necessary preparation for
Harvey's labours. Vesalius opened up the way for physiological inquiry by his exact anatomical labours but, as we have
seen, left the physiological plough almost as soon as he had
put his hand to it. And his successors did little more than
widen the way which he had opened up. Harvey was the first
who followed up the anatomical path till it led to a great
physiological truth.

Having made sure of the anatomical facts and having
grasped the suggestions which these offered, he proceeded at
once to test those suggestions by experiments on living
animals. It was, as he himself has said, through many vivisections that he was led to truth.

He made no appeal to any knowledge or to any conceptions
outside the facts of anatomy and the results of experiments.
Though few at that time could speak of the processes of living
bodies without bringing in the actions of spirits, natural, vital,
or animal, ever seeking to explain those processes by what the
spirits effected, Harvey left these spirits entirely on one side;
as we have seen, in one passage only in his book does he refer
to them, and then simply to dismiss them as irrelevant. On
the other hand he in like manner made no appeal, as the so-
called philosophers of his time and of times before had done, to
the general properties of matter, to the phenomena presented
by all things, whether living or not living. There is no
attempt in his book to solve the problems of the living body
by an appeal to what we now call physical and chemical laws.
His work, as I have said, is purely and strictly physiological.

And indeed when Harvey began his studies there was no exact science of physics or of chemistry to which he could appeal. There was plenty of philosophizing about nature and, as we shall see, the foundations of chemistry were being laid; but there was no sound body of truth which he could call in to his help. In one respect the science of living things was at this epoch ahead of that of things not alive, for the latter had no such solid basis as was already supplied to the former by anatomy.

During Harvey's lifetime however, even while he was labouring at his great work, an important change in this respect was taking place. During the early part of the seventeenth century the science of physics sprang into being, and a little later on rational chemistry began to emerge from a mystic alchemy. No sooner had these two sciences come to the front, than they were pressed sometimes wisely, sometimes unwisely into the science of physiology, sometimes wisely, to the great profit of physiology as an independent science, sometimes unwisely, whereby the school of physiology proper, the school of Vesalius and Harvey, was split up into the school of those who proposed to explain all the phenomena of the body and to cure all its ills on physical and mathematical principles, the iatro-mathematical or iatro-physical school, and into the school of those who proposed to explain all the same phenomena as mere chemical events, the iatro-chemical school.

When Harvey reached Padua in 1598, and conversed as he doubtless did with members of the University other than those who were studying, like himself, anatomy and medicine, he must have heard much of the man who had come to Padua from Pisa some six years before, and who making use and at the same time further developing a new method of thought and a new means of inquiry, which under the name of mathematics had been making great progress in the latter half of the preceding century, was bringing forth astounding new things, not only about the sun and the stars, but also about the working of machines and the fundamental properties of matter. For Galileo Galilei had in 1592 left his native city Pisa, where he had already made some of his immortal discoveries, to become Professor at Padua, where till 1610 he fruitfully laboured, as yet unharassed, for the blood-hounds of the Church had not caught scent of the heresies of his teachings.

It is not for me here to dwell on Galileo's labours in physical science; but it is important, in the history of physiology, to remember that through his and his fellow-labourers' inquiries, the science of physics made at this epoch a great bound forward. The influence of that progress made itself almost immediately felt in the science of living things.

Before I go on however to speak of the definite new contributions to physiology which may be regarded as the more or less direct outcome of the new school of exact and mathematical physical science, I must as it were turn aside to speak of one who without making so much as one single physiological discovery wrote a treatise on and expounded a complete system of physiology. This however he wrote not for the purpose of advancing physiology in particular, but as a contribution to a general system of philosophy; and though by it physiology gained no immediate new results, indeed much of the teaching contained in it was retrograde, yet the general ideas which inspired it influenced physiological thinkers even of his own time, and still more those of the times which followed.

René Descartes, born near Tours in 1596, and dying at Stockholm in 1650, makes a great figure in the history of human thought. He was a great mathematician; he may be said to have invented analytical geometry. He was an accomplished physicist; his theory of the Universe (*Le Monde*, 1664) influenced men's opinions about nature for many a year. Above all he was a philosopher. His *Discours de la Méthode*, 1637, made an epoch. But he was neither an anatomist nor a physiologist; he studied both anatomy and physiology, but not as an inquirer. He approached these matters as an amateur, but as an amateur having a special purpose, as one desirous to construct out of the current knowledge of the time a physiological basis for his philosophical views.

It was part of his philosophy to shew that man consisted of an earthly machine (*machine de terre*) inhabited and governed by a rational soul (*âme raisonnable*); and under the title of 'Man,' *L'Homme* (*De Homine Liber*, 1662), he wrote a treatise of physiology, not, as I have said, as a contribution to physiological knowledge, but as a popular exposition of the features of the earthly machine in illustration of its relations to the rational soul. The work thus stands out as the first Text-Book of Physiology, written after the modern fashion, though in a popular way. We may perhaps speak of him as the Herbert Spencer of the age in so far that his treatise on man bore somewhat the same relation to the physiological inquiries of the time as the Principles of Biology do to the biological researches of the present day.

But Descartes had much more distinctly in view than had Spencer the object of popular exposition, and he had especially in view the exposition of the mode of action of the soul. Thus though he begins with the beginning, namely with the ingestion of food, he hurries over digestion and also over the circulation. He was acquainted with Harvey's work, but he had not been convinced by Harvey's arguments; he was not familiar enough with the details of physiological inquiry to feel the full force of Harvey's reasonings. He admitted Harvey's great and new conclusion, the greater circulation, the passage of blood from the arteries to the veins, but he would not admit what Harvey insisted, and truly insisted upon as the keystone of his whole argument, the propulsion of the blood by the systole, by the contraction of the heart. He clung in the main to the old doctrines. This is what he says:

After speaking of the formation of blood in the liver out of the chyle of the food, he goes on thus,

"Now this blood has one obvious passage only by which it "can get out, namely that one which carries it into the right "cavity of the heart; and you must know that the tissue of "the heart contains in its pores one of those fires without light "of which I spoke above, which makes it so hot, so ardent "that no sooner does the blood enter into one or other of the "two chambers or cavities which are in the heart, than it "immediately expands and dilates, just as you would find the "blood or the milk of an animal would do if you were to pour "it drop by drop into a vessel which was very hot. And the "fire which exists in the heart of the machine which I am "describing serves no other purpose than that of expanding, "heating and as it were subtilizing the blood which falls

"continually drop by drop, through the channel of the vena
"cava into the cavity of its right side, whence it is exhaled into
"the lung, and from the vein of the lung, which the anatomists
"call the vein-like artery, into the cavity of the other side,
"whence it is distributed over the whole body.

"The tissue of the lung is so delicate and soft and always
"kept so fresh by the air breathed that so soon as the vapours
"of the blood which pass out from the right cavity of the heart
"enter into the artery which the anatomists call the artery-
"like vein, they are condensed and converted once more into
"blood, and then fall drop by drop into the left cavity of the
"heart, where if they entered without being condensed anew
"they would not be adequate to nourish the fire which exists
"there.

*   *   *   *   *   *   *

"The pulse or beating of the arteries depends on eleven
"little membranes which like so many little doors open and
"close the openings of the four vessels which open into the
"two cavities of the heart. For at the moment that one of the
"beats ceases and another is ready to begin, the little doors
"attached to the openings of the two arteries are firmly closed
"while those at the openings of the two veins remain open, so
"that two drops of blood cannot help falling by these two
"veins, one into each cavity of the heart. These drops of
"blood are then rarified, and all of a sudden filling up a space
"incomparably greater than that which they occupied before,
"press upon and close those little doors which guard the
"entrances to the veins, preventing by this means any more
"blood falling into the heart, and press upon and open the
"doors of the two arteries, into which they, the drops of blood,
"enter promptly and with force, thus making the heart and
"with it all the arteries of the body expand. But immediately
"afterwards this rarified blood is condensed once more or
"penetrates into other parts; and thus the heart and arteries
"cease to be distended, the little doors which guard the en-
"trances to the two arteries close again, and those which guard
"the entrances to the two veins open again and give passage
"to two other drops of blood, which once more make the heart
"and arteries expand, just like those which went before."

Such is Descartes' dogmatic exposition of the working of the heart. Rejecting Harvey's new conclusions, he takes his stand on the old Galenic doctrine of the innate heat of the heart, and of the expansion of the heart by that heat. But indeed about these things he did not care much; his mind was set on the nervous system; he was concerned with the circulation only so far as this supplied the material basis of nervous energy. He only sought to explain how the blood, itself derived from the food, gave rise to those animal spirits by means of which the special earthly machine, the brain with its nerves, carried out the behests of the rational soul. He thus explains how the best part of the blood is carried to the brain for the purpose of generating the animal spirits:

"The most agitated and vivified parts of the blood, being "carried to the brain by the arteries which spring from the "heart in the most direct line, constitute as it were a very "subtle air or wind, called the animal spirits, which dilating "the brain fit it to receive the impressions of external objects "and also those of the soul, that is to say, fit it to be the seat "of common sensation, of imagination, and of memory. This "air or these spirits then flow from the brain along the nerves "into all the muscles, whereby they dispose the nerves to "serve as the organs of the external senses, and finally "distending the muscles give movement to all the limbs."

What I have just quoted is enough to shew that Descartes was not a physiological inquirer. His method in physiology was not that of Harvey, not that which since Harvey's time has continued to bring in a rich harvest of discovered truth, not that of working one's way by careful observation, and patient experiment or trial, out of exactly determined anatomical facts, up to the real meaning of the facts. He had a special purpose in view, and with that in view took a freer, wider sweep. He had to shew that the new views which were making it clear in so surprising a way that the universe was a machine working in accordance with physical laws, might be applied also to man; that man, that is to say the body of man, might also be regarded as a machine working in accordance with physical laws. He had to shew this with the help of the knowledge of the time, and he achieved this by picking out such parts of the anatomical discoveries of the age as suited his purpose, and by weaving these together with many other statements, for which he gives no authority and which he yet treats as accredited truths, into a theory of the constitution and action of the nervous system viewed as a mere machine.

I shall have occasion in a later lecture to dwell on some of the details of Descartes' theory of the working of the nervous system, and to shew how he utilized the doctrine of the animal spirits to explain the phenomena of sensation and movement. For him, as we shall see, the animal spirits constituted a fluid, a very subtle fluid it is true, but still a fluid amenable to the physical laws governing fluids, and for him the nerves were tubes along which the spirits flowed in a wholly mechanical manner. In his exposition he makes assumptions, such as the presence in the nerves of valvular arrangements, for which he gives no evidence and for which he had no authority. I do not enter into these points now, I only wish to call attention to his work as an attempt to apply the new philosophy of exact mathematics and physics to the interpretation of the phenomena of living things.

Descartes' contemporaries stumbled, as we now stumble, at those parts of the basis of his views for which they could find no authority given by anatomical observation or by physiological experiment. Hence his views on the nature of man found no place in the physiology of the day, they passed over wholly into philosophy so called. But his main idea, that the problems of man ought to be treated in the same way as the problems of the rest of nature, made itself felt and produced effects in after times.

I cannot do better than quote the words of a remarkable contemporary of his, one of whom I shall soon have to speak, Nicolas Stensen, who in a discourse delivered in Paris on the anatomy of the brain thus sums up Descartes' position as a physiologist.

"Descartes," says he, "was too clever in exposing the errors "of current treatises on man to be willing to undertake the "task of expounding the true structure of man. Therefore in "his essay on Man he does not attempt such a delineation, but "is content to describe a machine capable of performing all

"the functions of which man is capable. And in this sense we
"may affirm without exaggeration that Descartes bears the
"palm over all other philosophers in this matter. For he was
"the first who dared to explain all the functions of man, and
"especially of the brain, in a mechanical manner. Other
"authors describe man; Descartes puts before us merely a
"machine, but by means of this he very clearly exposed the
"ignorance of others who have treated of man, and opened up
"for us a way by which to investigate the use of other parts
"of the body, though it may be difficult to do so with the same
"clearness and fidelity with which he proceeds in demon-
"strating the parts of his machine of man, a task which no
"man before him attempted."

From this excursion into wider fields we now return to the
narrower one of the effects of the teaching of Galileo on the
more special problems of physiology, and this brings us at once
to the labours of Borelli.

Giovanni Alphonso Borelli was born at Naples on Jan. 28,
1608, in the Nuovo Castello, where his father, a man of humble
origin, though his mother was of a good family, was serving as
a soldier. Of his early days little or nothing is known, but he
himself tells us that he studied mathematics at Rome under
Benedetto Castello. His great ability was not only at once
obvious to his teacher but soon became known to others; for
while as yet a young man, probably about 1640 or possibly
earlier, he was invited to and accepted the Chair of Mathematics at the University of Messina, which was then making
itself felt as an active seat of learning. He, like other mathe-
maticians of the time, was a pupil of Galileo, in the sense that
he had learnt much from that great man through his writings
and indirectly in other ways. But he had apparently never
listened to his voice, and so earnestly did he desire to do so
that with the consent and indeed at the expense of the
University he left Messina for a while in order to visit Florence
and see Galileo. Unhappily very soon after his arrival in 1642
Galileo died, and Borelli, though he appears to have stayed
some time in Florence enjoying intercourse with Torricelli,
returned to Messina, where in 1649 he published his first work,
an account of the pestilence raging in Sicily in 1647–8. Though

in the first place a mathematician and a physicist, he like other learned men of the time busied himself with inquiries reaching outside his own line; that he was justified in doing so is shewn by the fact that in this treatise he attacked the views held by physicians concerning the cause of the disease, and contended that it was due to what we should now call an air-borne germ.

His fame while at Messina grew so great and spread so far that in 1656 he was invited by Ferdinand Duke of Tuscany to fill the Chair of Mathematics in the University of Pisa. The efforts of the Medici to make their university an academic power were being crowned with success, and Pisa was now outshining Padua. Borelli accepted the invitation, and so began what was perhaps the brightest and the best part of his career, though he was already forty-eight years old.

Much as he owed to his chief teacher Castello, Borelli was to a large extent a self-taught man. He seems not to have paid much attention to literary studies, and his life at Messina was probably more or less a provincial life, a life marked with provincial characters. Coming to Pisa he was plunged at once into the most polished life of the times. And there is a story that at the introductory lecture, which against his will he was induced to give upon entering into office, his clumsy diction, his rude gestures, his long-winded and yet halting sentences were so little to the taste of his fastidious audience that they broke out into derisive laughter and brought the lecture to a premature close.

In spite of this Borelli soon made his power felt. Though his chief duty was to teach mathematics, he threw himself with zeal also into other kinds of learning. Malpighi, as we shall presently see, came from Bologna to Pisa at the close of the year of Borelli's arrival. The two at once became close friends, and anatomy soon occupied Borelli's energies almost as much as mathematics and physics. By his talents and energy he made the University of Pisa famous as a school for both mathematical and medical science, and his efforts in these directions were generously supported by the munificence of the Medici. It was perhaps chiefly through Borelli's unwearied activity in advancing by way of experiment natural knowledge of all kinds that in 1657, under the patronage of Prince Leopold, the famous Academia del Cimento, one of the first of learned societies, was instituted. Borelli, Malpighi, and the sagacious naturalist Redi formed a trio which would have been an ornament to any academy. But the Cimento was not all union. Borelli's intellectual gifts lacked the support of an amiable character; he was morose and quarrelsome, tenacious of his own right, not unenvious of the success of others, and apt when contradicted or opposed to fly into a passion; some of his contemporaries speak of him as almost unbearable. He was more than once led into a quarrel with his colleagues of the Academy, and eventually became estranged even from Malpighi, who looked upon him as a father, and who while they were at Pisa together sought counsel of him almost every day.

During these years Borelli published not only mathematical works, such as his *Euclides restitutus*, and astronomical works, for at Florence during the summer when freed from the duty of lecturing he under the patronage of the Medici made observations on the heavens, but also his important physical work, *De vi percussionis*. But what he set his mind chiefly to do was to write a treatise on animal motion, *De motu animalium*, embodying the results of the anatomical and physiological inquiries in which he had been so long engaged, and to the prosecution of which he had so fruitfully stimulated others. Although the work was not to see the light for many years, much of it apparently was written before he left Pisa.

For he did leave Pisa. It seems strange that he should desire to leave such a centre of light to live once more in an out of the way and provincial seat of learning. He pleaded as his reasons the ungenial climate of Pisa and the desire for more leisure and quiet; others thought it was his inconstant temper and his repeated quarrels with his colleagues that led him, in 1668, after twelve years' stay at Pisa to accept an invitation to return to his old University at Messina. Here, if he had more leisure, his intellectual activity at least in spite of his increasing years shewed no signs of being on the wane. He published his important treatise on 'The natural movements depending on gravity,' he investigated an eruption of Etna, he busied himself in literary and antiquarian studies and all the while he continued working on what he felt to be his great effort, the treatise on animal motion.

In 1674, being concerned, or being suspected of being concerned, in a political conspiracy to free Sicily from the rule of Spain, he left Messina for the last time and fled an exile to Rome. There was at that time living in Rome that remarkable, I ought perhaps to say notorious, woman Christina (daughter of Gustavus Adolphus of Sweden), who after bearing the burdens of the crown for ten years (for at her father's death in 1644 she succeeded to the throne) threw them on one side in 1654, in order that, free from political cares, she might devote herself to the charms of travel and of intellectual culture, and to other pleasures of private life. She, playing the part of Lady Bountiful in science, held a little academy of her own, and when Borelli, a needy, or well-nigh needy, exile arrived at Rome, she took him under her protection. He earned the assistance which she gave him by acting as her physician and also by frequently delivering discourses at her academy, discourses which however he did not think worthy of being published. For three years he continued thus under her patronage, though living in his own house on the slender means which he still retained and on the help which she gave him. He kept on labouring at his book on animal motion, the expenses of the publication of which Christina undertook to defray; and in 1676 the work was so near completion that Borelli felt justified in writing the dedication to her.

The pecuniary aid which Borelli received from Queen Christina was somewhat uncertain, owing to the fitful way in which her remittances arrived from Sweden. In 1677 a heavy blow fell upon him; his private servant robbed him of all his little money, and indeed all his property; and need led him to take up his abode among the Society of the Scholae Piae of San Pantaleone, where he dwelt for two years, giving the penultimate touches to his great work, which as he said he had promised to the world twenty-four years before, and earning his board and lodging by teaching mathematics to the young scholars of the society. The last touches which were needed he did not live to give; before the book had left the press he was seized with a pleurisy, and on the last day of 1679, just as the new year was coming in, he passed away. The pupil of Galileo, like his master, bowed before the power of the Church, and an ecclesiastic dignitary, writing the preface to the work of Borelli, published the year after his death, breaks out into praises of the pious life of the great man of science, especially commending him in that when in his lectures on astronomy he had to speak of 'systems' he maintained the authority of the Church. "Whatever others may have taught, it is our "duty, he used to say, not to listen to it. As the Holy Church "teaches so ought we to believe, and obeying her, to hold as "true whatever she lays down."

Borelli was essentially a mathematician and a physicist; of his valuable contributions to these sciences this is not the place to speak. The problems of the living body were not to him, as they had been to Vesalius and Harvey, the object of a first love. Their care had been to find an answer to the biological question; and they used all other knowledge as a means to this end. He, on the other hand, regarded the phenomena presented by living beings as a field yielding him abundant opportunities for applying the new methods of physical research. And we cannot wonder that from this point of view the movements of animals early attracted his attention. As we have just said, his great work, *De motu animalium*, was not published until after his death, the first volume appearing in 1680, the second in 1681; but as we have also said, what is printed in them had been taught publicly long before, while he was as yet professor in Pisa; and indeed much of the work must have been already in manuscript in those early years, for his pupil Bellini, writing in 1662, refers to it as already a book.

He himself makes quite clear his own opinion of the real nature of his book. In the introduction he speaks of physiology, a word which employed rarely in earlier times, by Aselli for instance, was now coming into general use as a 'part of physics,' and this he proposes 'to ornament and enrich by mathematical demonstrations.'

Animal movements naturally divide themselves into external movements, such as those effected by the skeletal muscles, and internal movements, such as the movements of the heart and of other viscera, and in general the movements of the fluid parts of the body. Borelli treats of each. We will consider the external movements first.

The various movements effected by the muscles present two classes of problems: the special problems, mechanical in nature, of the movements effected by particular muscles; and the more general problem, in a certain sense also a physical one, how the substance of a muscle gives rise to movement, by what changes in a muscle movement is brought about.

A large part of Borelli's work is devoted to the special mechanical problems. Vesalius, and later on Fabricius, had treated of these problems in some detail, but they had treated of them in a more or less loose way only. They lacked, Vesalius wholly, and Fabricius to a less but still to a great extent, the exact mathematical and mechanical knowledge which springing up in the latter part of the sixteenth century made such rapid progress in the beginning of the seventeenth century under Galileo and his school. Borelli was of that school, and having laid a foundation in a chapter entitled, 'Mechanical propositions useful for the more exact determination of the motive power of muscles,' he treats in succession of the various problems of muscular mechanics, of flexion and extension, and of the more complex problems of standing, walking, running, and other forms of locomotion; he investigates these in the same rigid, exact manner, calling in the aid of mathematical figures and calculations, as he and others had investigated the problems of falling bodies, and of the action of various propulsive and other machines.

One has only to compare the chapters of Fabricius with those of Borelli which deal with any one of these problems, that of walking for instance, in order to realize what a large bound forward mechanical science had made in the first years of the seventeenth century.

Borelli's discussions concerning these special problems may be read with profit even at the present day; they supply the basis of muscular mechanics, and interspersed among them will be found shrewd observations, which pass from mere mechanics into more distinctly physiological questions, such for instance as that in which he calls attention to the distinction between the weak tonic contraction which a muscle may exercise against an antagonist muscle, and the more powerful voluntary contraction by which the same muscle does work equivalent to raising a heavy weight.

Not content with the solution of these problems of muscular mechanics, problems which could be solved by the almost direct application of known mechanical methods, and which called for little special research beyond the mere determination of the necessary data, Borelli passes on to the more general, more distinctly physiological, far more difficult question of the nature of muscular movement; this also he attempts to solve by the mechanical mathematical method.

It was recognized of old that the movements of the limbs and of the various parts of the body were brought about by the shortening of the structures called muscles. It was also recognized that nerves were concerned in the action, it being generally supposed that animal spirits passing along the nerves to the muscle provoked in some way or other the movement. In the muscle itself two parts were recognized: the fibres of the muscle which, though possessing a nature of their own, passed into and were continuous with the fibres of the tendon at each end, and the flesh, 'caro,' which filled up the interstices between the fibres and adapted itself to them, but which otherwise was comparable with the flesh, 'caro,' or parenchyma of other organs, such for instance as the liver. According at least to general opinion, the contraction, that is the shortening and hardening of the muscle as a whole, was carried out not by the flesh, 'caro,' but by the fibres of the muscle, the power of the fibres to effect this being due to the animal spirits reaching them along the nerves.

Vesalius, passing lightly over this, as over other problems distinctly physiological rather than anatomical, and this as we have seen was his wont, has little to say about it, but that little goes straight to the root of the matter. He saw clearly that the contractile power of the muscle resides in the actual muscular substance, not in the fibres of the ligament or tendon which spread out into the muscle's belly, nor in the nerves distributed in it, though these played their part as carriers of the animal spirits. This is what he says:

"Muscle therefore, which is the instrument of voluntary "movement as the eye is the instrument of vision and the "tongue of taste, is composed of the substance of the ligament "or tendon divided into a great number of fibres and of flesh "containing and embracing these fibres. It also receives "branches of arteries, veins and nerves, and by reason of "the presence of the nerves is never destitute of animal "spirits so long as the animal is sound and well. Now I do "not regard this flesh as merely a foundation or basis, as it "were a bed or support by which the fibres and the above-"mentioned divisions of the nerves are held together. Nor "do I with Plato and Aristotle (who did not at all understand "the nature of muscle) attribute to the flesh so slight a duty "as to serve, after the fashion of fat or grease or some sort "of clothing, the purpose of lessening the effects of heat in "summer and of cold in winter. On the contrary, I am per-"suaded that the flesh of muscles, which is different from "everything else in the whole body, is the chief agent, by aid "of which (the nerves, the messengers of the animal spirits "not being wanting) the muscle becomes thicker, shortens "and gathers itself together, and so draws to itself and moves "the part to which it is attached, and by help of which it again "relaxes and extends, and so lets go again the part which it "had so drawn. It is clear that the proper substance of an "organ is the agent of the primary functions of the organ, as "is the case in the brain, heart, liver, lungs, spleen, kidney "and testes."

Fabricius discourses in three long rambling chapters on the structure, the action, and the uses of muscle. In these he shews here and there the influence of new ideas, as for instance when he compares the action of a nerve in inducing muscular contraction, though itself not contracting, to that of a magnet which causes a piece of iron to move, though not itself moving. Yet his teaching is on the whole the old teach-ing that the contractile power resides in the fibres of the muscle, not in the flesh. So far from advancing beyond Vesalius, he falls behind him; in this as in other matters Galen is his master, not Vesalius. Indeed when Borelli attacked the problem, this was very much where Vesalius had left it, for Descartes had passed it lightly over.

He had the advantage of being able to start with a truer knowledge of the minute structure of muscle. As we shall see in the succeeding lecture the microscope had about this time come to the aid of the anatomist, and Malpighi, Borelli's friend and colleague at Pisa, was using the new aid as a means of achieving brilliant discoveries concerning the finer structure of living beings. Nor was the new instrument being used by anatomists at Pisa only. Before Borelli's book was published, but, probably, not before he had written or at least begun to write it, there appeared in 1664 a little tract, *De musculis observationum specimen*, expanded and illustrated with figures a few years later in 1667 as *Elementorum myologiae specimen*, written by a Dane, Nicolas Stensen, better known perhaps by his Latin name of Steno, to whom I have already referred and of whom I will venture to say something more in detail in a succeeding lecture. Stensen had used the microscope and had been led to the following conception of the structure of a muscle.

According to him a muscle is essentially a collection of motor fibres. Each motor fibre (*fibra motrix*), itself a complex of most minute fibrils, arranged lengthways, has a middle part, which differs in consistency, thickness and colour from each of the ends. The several motor fibres are bound together by the continuous transverse fibrillae of the proper membrane of the muscle. The middle parts of the motor fibres, wrapped round by the membranous fibrillae, constitute together the fleshy part of the muscle, which soft, broad and thick differs in colour in different animals, being reddish or pale or even whitish; in the leg of the rabbit you will find some muscles red and others pale. The end parts of the motor fibres, which are always white, thin, and tough, constitute together the tendons. It is the fleshy parts of the motor fibres and these alone which contract, and in doing so become shorter, harder, and corrugated on the surface; the tendinous parts remain unchanged.

It will be seen that Stensen had come very near to a true conception of the structure of muscle. What he called a 'motor fibre' we now call a 'fasciculus,' his 'most minute fibril' is our 'elementary fibre,' and we speak of his 'proper membrane' with its transverse fibrillae as 'the connective tissue framework.' Stensen too, like Borelli, was full of the new spirit of the mechanical philosophy of the day; and the greater part of the work of which I am speaking is taken up with elaborate mathematical mechanical expositions. In a muscle, says Stensen, the middle fleshy part is an oblique-angled parallelepiped, and the tendon at each end is a tetragonal prism; and he develops at length the geometrical consequences of this conception.

Borelli was acquainted with Stensen's work, he accepts his exposition of the structure of muscle, and speaks of muscular fibres and muscular fasciculi as the real contractile part, the fibres of the tendon serving only to bind the fleshy fibres to bones or other structures. It is true that he refutes Stensen's mathematical mechanical conceptions of the arrangement of the fibres, replacing them by conceptions of his own; but this is a matter of little moment. Both observers had grasped the all-important fundamental fact that the act of contraction is carried out by the fleshy muscular fibre and that the fibres of the tendon, howsoever far they may seem to enter the muscle, are mere passive agents, retaining their normal length and consistence and taking no part whatever in the contraction. The old idea of the contractile tendinous fibres, and of the flesh 'caro,' serving the purpose of mere packing was done away with for ever, and Vesalius was justified of his children.

Coming then to the actual nature of this contraction of the fleshy part, Borelli strove very hard to reach a definite mechanical explanation of the process. In this he, in one respect, went distinctly astray. Recognizing the beat of the heart as a contraction of the muscular ventricles, and impressed with the fact that during the systole the walls of the ventricles closing in laterally obliterate the cavities from which the blood has been driven, he concluded that the muscular walls in contracting increase in bulk; and he extended this conclusion to all muscles. This view of an increase in bulk led him to suppose that the hardening and tension observable when a muscle contracts is due, not to mere displacement of the parts of the muscle itself, but to an inflation of the muscular substance by something from without. And in accordance with this he constructs a hypothesis, in which the muscular fibres are supposed to be chains of rhombs, and proceeds to shew how contraction, with its attendant hardening and extension, may be explained by considering inflation as being the sudden insertion of a number of wedges.

Having reached this mechanical conception of the act of contraction itself, he attempts to gain a like mechanical conception of the way in which the nerves act as the exciting agents of this contraction. He begins his discussion of the subject by refuting the wrong explanations of muscular contraction which had been put forward by various authors.

"Although Nature is admirable in all her operations, yet "there is no one who is not in the highest degree astounded "when he considers the immense force and energy of muscles, "and sets about to understand more exactly the causes, "organs and apparatus by which Nature carries out such a "work. And for the reason that human stupidity is more "easily struck with the ugliness of error than with the beauty "of truth, I shall first proceed to expose wrong views, both "because this part of science is not to be despised, and also "because the exclusion of what is erroneous the more easily "leads us to the discovery of what is true."

The first wrong view which he exposes is the one that muscles are directly moved by some incorporeal agency.

"Muscles do not exercise vital movement otherwise than "by contracting. Such a violent contraction however is not "brought about by anything else than the hardening and "inflation which the muscle undergoes. Now such an inflation "cannot be conceived without the advent and insinuation of "a second body. For the corporeal mass of the muscle, "possessing as it does three dimensions, cannot be inflated "and increased in bulk by any wholly incorporeal influence "having like an indivisible point no magnitude."

He next refutes the view that muscular movement is brought about by spirits or by a corporeal air, such as the atmosphere is.

"There are not wanting those who insist that extremely "attenuated corporeal animal spirits like air supply the cause "of the movements of muscles.

"But these cannot extricate themselves from innumerable "difficulties. For, according to their views that spirituous air "either expands the muscles, rushing into their cavities like "wind, and filling them with its abundance and plenty, or on "the other hand brings about the contraction by filling up the "porosities of the muscles through ebullition and rarefaction. "But this seems to be impossible because the action of a "muscle is a mere contraction of its length, so that the two "ends by contrary movements are brought towards each "other, the muscle swelling and enlarging in breadth."

After pointing out the various difficulties he says, "Finally "a very common experiment does away with all this nonsense "about air. When the muscles of a living animal are divided "lengthwise, while the animal is submerged under water, and "in consequence of the pain is struggling violently, in the "midst of such great copious fervour and ebullition of the "supposed spirituous gas which would thereby be excited in "the muscles, one would expect that innumerable bubbles "of gas would burst forth from the wound, and ascend "through the water, whereas nothing of the kind takes "place."

He further goes on to shew that vital contraction cannot take place by reason of any juice or blood distending the porosities of the muscles, nor from the blood being driven into them by the force of the heart.

Having thus discussed the wrong explanations, he proceeds to expound the probably true explanation of muscular contraction.

He concludes that for bringing about muscular contraction two causes are necessary, one existing in the muscle itself, the other brought to it from without.

"Since all muscles, with some few exceptions, do not "manifest vital movement otherwise than in obedience to the "will, since the commands of the will are not transmitted from "the brain which is the instrument of the sensitive, and the "seat of the motive soul, by any other channels than the

"nerves as all confess and as the most decided experiments
"shew, and since the action of any incorporeal agency or of
"spirituous gases must be rejected, it is clear that some cor
"poreal substance must be transmitted along the nerves to
"the muscles or else some commotion must be communicated
"along some substance in the nerves, in such a way that a
"very powerful inflation can be brought about in the twink-
"ling of an eye.

"And since the inflation, hardening, and contraction do
"not take place in the channels which serve for bringing them
"about and in which the motor influence resides, namely, in
"the nerves themselves, but takes place outside the nerves,
"namely, in the muscles, it is evident that the substance or
"the influence which the nerves transmit is not taken by itself
"alone sufficient to bring about that inflation. It is necessary,
"therefore, that something else must be added, something
"which is to be found in the muscles themselves; or that in
"the muscles there is some adequate disposition of material
"so that on the arrival of the influence transmitted by the
"nerves there takes place something like a fermentation or
"ebullition, by which the sudden inflation of the muscle is
"brought about. That such an action is possible is rendered
"clear by innumerable experiments which are continually
"being made in chemical elaborations as when spirits of vitriol
"are poured on oil of tartar; indeed all acid spirits when mixed
"with fixed salts at once boil up with a sudden fermentation.
"In like manner, therefore, we may suppose that there takes
"place in a muscle a somewhat similar mixing from which a
"sudden fermentation and ebullition results, with the mass
"of which the porosities of the muscle are filled up and
"enlarged, thus bringing about the turgescence and the
"inflation."

I must not dwell any longer on Borelli's views concerning
muscular contraction. I shall have to take them up again in
connection with the labours of other men on the same subject.
I have said enough to shew how great and rapid an advance
in our knowledge of these matters had been brought about by
the new physical learning. Working on mechanical mathematical lines, and almost on these alone—for it is only at the

end that he calls to his aid some of the chemical ideas which were beginning to stir men's minds, and his no less than others, but which were as yet far behind the already current physical ideas—Borelli was able to approach very near the conception which was not to be laid hold of for a century or more, the conception of the irritability of muscle maintained by nutritive processes, and of the calling that irritability into play by the advent of nervous impulses.

Borelli had also much to say concerning the internal movements of the body, movements other than those carried out by the skeletal muscles. He dwells at length on the movements of the heart and on the circulation.

He fully accepts Harvey's views, and develops them in his own way. Although Harvey could not be ignorant of the exact mathematical and physical knowledge which was being gathered up in his time, he as we have seen makes little or no use of it in his great work. That was based exclusively on the teachings of anatomy and the results of experiments on living animals; he never made use of the new mathematical or even the new physical methods. This is exactly what Borelli does. To the physicist the problems of the circulation have always been fascinating; they obviously were so to Borelli, and he develops a number of mechanical investigations and specula-- tions. While his brother-mathematician Descartes was content with the old view of the expansion of the ventricles by the rarefaction and dilatation of the contents through the innate heat, Borelli seizes the Harveian view of the propulsive power of the heart in its systole and likens the ventricle to a wine-press or to a piston. He dwells on the mechanical action of the spiral arrangement of the fibres of the ventricle, an arrangement which he says he himself had discovered, though there is reason to think that the observation is due to Malpighi, and speaks of the work done by the heart in the following terms:

"The true action of the muscle of the heart is the contrac-"tion of its ventricles, and the compression and expression of "the blood contained in them is carried out after the manner "of a winepress, and that not by the contortion of the spiral "fibres of the heart but by their inflation and tension."

He gives the following as the reason why the lateral walls of the heart are brought together in the systole:

"All the almost innumerable fibres are carried obliquely "and transversely round the sides of the heart, and form a "number of strata placed one upon the other like a series of "membranes. When therefore the fibres of any stratum are "inflated, these touching each other laterally and lying in one "plane naturally push each other sideways, and so mutually "shove each other out of their proper places, and push each "other away from their proper situation, namely towards the "base and the apex. This would tend to increase the interval "between the base and the apex; but other external fibres "surrounding the obliquely transverse ones and intersecting "them in a decussating manner prevent, as we shall presently "shew, their elongation and protuberance, whence necessarily "the inflation of those fibres gives rise to an intumescence "internally towards the cavities and so the inflated internal "sides of the walls are brought nearer to each other."

We have seen that an important link in Harvey's argument was furnished by his calculations as to the quantity of blood driven into the arteries from the heart, calculations which were as we shall see repeated in a more exact manner some years later by Richard Lower. Borelli goes further, he is anxious to determine in mechanical terms the force of the ventricular systole. Assuming that the force of contraction of all healthy muscular tissue is the same for a unit of bulk, and observing that the 'fleshy mass of the heart' is in bulk equal to a masseter and temporal muscle combined, he concludes that it exercises the same force as these two together, which force can be determined experimentally. He finds that the muscles of the two sides of the jaw acting together can support a weight of more than 300 lbs. The muscles of one side therefore will support a weight of more than 150 lbs. But this is an instance of the partial force of a muscle; if we want to find the whole force of the muscle we ought to multiply this result at least 20 times. Thus he reaches the conclusion that the motive force of the heart considered by itself may be calculated as equal to that of supporting a weight of more than 3000 lbs.

Perhaps the most interesting part of Borelli's work on the circulation is his treatment of the flow in the arteries. Working on the lines of his view that the action of the heart is to be likened to the action of a piston in a pump, he argues that at the close of a heart-beat the arteries are not empty, but still hold a considerable quantity of blood; according to his calculations they contain about ¼ of the total blood of the body, the quantity introduced at a single beat, namely about three ounces, being a twentieth part of that, and occupying a space in the arteries next to the heart not more than half a foot in length.

He discusses at length the resistance which the heart has to overcome, resistance offered by the walls of the arteries themselves, by the tissues surrounding them, and by the minute and variously shaped orifices through which the blood issues from the terminations of the arteries in the several tissues. And by a series of mathematical calculations he comes to the conclusion that the heart in maintaining the circulation has at each beat to exert a force equivalent to not less than 135,000 lbs.

His view of the flow in the arteries is worth giving in his own words:

"In the first place we must disprove the common assertion "that blood is driven through the terminal orifices of the "arteries after the fashion of a fountain, simply by the pro-"pulsive force of the heart.

"The arteries are soft, distensible tubes full of blood, but as "we have shewn not filled to extreme distension; and during "each beat of the heart there is driven into them by the con-"striction of the heart, acting like a piston, a mass of blood "sufficient to complete their distension or even more than "sufficient, in which case the surplus is discharged beyond "the arteries by the beat of the heart itself. But so soon "as the beat is over the arteries return from their distended "condition to the same soft and shrunken state in which they "were before the beat. Therefore there must have escaped "from them the mass of blood or the surplus of that mass "which had been driven into them by the piston of the heart. "But the blood which has been driven into the arteries cannot

"issue from them of its own accord through the extremely
"minute terminal orifices of the arteries since it possesses no
"force of its own. Nor is it driven out by the propulsion of
"the piston of the heart or only partly so since the arteries are
"not rigid tubes made of steel but are soft, and the force of
"the heart in its direct action is spent in expanding them,
"which expansion acts as a cause of retention rather than of
"expulsion of the blood."

After shewing that the flow of blood out of the arteries
cannot be due to gravity, or to any force supplied by a
rarefaction of the blood, he goes on:

"Two effects follow the beat of the heart, the filling of the
"arteries with the blood driven into them, and the exit of the
"same blood from the same arteries. Certainly these two
"events cannot take place at the same time; for the one
"consists in an expansion, the other in a constriction of the
"same arteries, and these two being opposed in nature cannot
"take place at the same time. Whence it must be that the
"filling of the arteries takes place first, and that their con-
"striction and emptying follows afterwards.

"The filling and distension however which take place first
"cannot be carried out without a violent extension of the
"transverse fibres of the said arteries. Now we know from
"other sources that all fibres of vessels, and all fibres of
"muscles, of the intestines, of tendons, of membrane, and of
"the true skin resist extension, and when extended possess
"a power of contracting like that of a strung bow. Nay,
"indeed, we see that all fibres when placed in their natural
"surroundings possess some amount of active tension, for
"when they are divided they contract of their own accord
"and become shorter. This would not happen if these fibres
"existed in a condition of equilibrium between extension and
"contraction; like the cord of an unstrung bow they would
"suffer neither contraction nor extension.

"But if all fibres in a natural condition undergo some
"amount of extension it follows that, when the arteries are
"filled with blood, the transverse fibres, owing to the enlarge-
"ment of the cavity, must become much more elongated and
"in consequence undergo a much greater extension. And

"since the said expansion of the arteries is succeeded by a
"constriction which cannot take place without a shortening
"of the circular fibres, and indeed such a shortening is proper
"to and part of the very nature of these fibres, it follows that
"the arteries after their violent expansion, due to their being
"filled to distension, cannot do other than exercise by the
"law of nature that mechanical force which they possess. This
"squeezing the arteries like a rope twisted circularly round
"them expels with force the blood through their terminal
"orifices."

This has only to be translated into present language in
order to be read as stating that the steady flow from the
arteries through the capillaries into the veins is the result of
the elastic reactions of the arterial walls, and thus the indirect, not the direct, result of the heart-beat.

Some of Borelli's numerical calculations were misleading,
but even in quite recent times numerical calculations of
muscular force based on the latest researches have also proved
misleading, and such miscalculations in nowise lessen the
admiration which one must feel for work shewing, in such
early times after Harvey, such a grip of the problems of
haemodynamics. We may almost say, even not forgetting
Hales, that Borelli brought our knowledge of the subject
nearly to the point at which after the lapse of more than a
century, indeed of nearly two centuries, Poiseuille and Weber
took it up again.

Borelli completes his treatise on the circulation by considerations on the nature and cause of the heart-beat. In its
immediate nature the heart-beat, the movement of the heart,
is identical with the movement of a limb; both are muscular
contractions of the same order. But the two differ in their ultimate cause. The movement of the limb is the issue of a direct
action of the will, the movement of the heart is not so. "It may
"arise by organic necessity, the heart may move as certain
"automata move. Or possibly the movement may come from
"a voluntary effort of which we have ceased to be conscious
"because it has been repeated so often and so constantly."

After treating the movements of the circulation thus fully,
Borelli goes on to attack by similar methods the problems of

respiration. Of his views on this subject I will not speak here; it will be convenient to deal with them in another connection. Nor did he stop at respiration. As we shall see in the next lecture physiologists were becoming much exercised in their minds concerning the structure of glands and the nature of the process of secretion. Borelli attacked these problems also, and satisfied himself that all the phenomena of secretion could be explained in a mechanical manner by the help of hypotheses concerning the size and shape of the particles to be secreted, and of the orifices or spaces through which they had to pass. This is what he says:

"For we have shewn that the fluidity of a liquid cannot be "conceived of without its mass being actually divisible into "very minute hard and consistent particles of a definite shape, "united together not by firm bonds but by simple contact, so "that some of them can be agitated, can flow, can move about "while others are at rest or are moving in another direction. "In no other way can be preserved that fluidity through "which fluid parts flow along, mix and fuse together.

"Moreover it cannot be doubted that the different natures "and properties of fluids depend on the different consistency, "structure, configuration and motion of the molecules com-"posing the fluids. Thus the molecules composing water are "all homogeneous and like each other but different from those "composing oil or a fluid of another nature, and indeed it is "agreed that the particles of the said fluids differ in structure, "size and shape.

"And indeed if the molecules of two heterogeneous fluids "were equally mobile so that they could be mixed by simple "contact, then a mixture of them, a mixture for instance of "oil and water, might be compared to a mixed heap of millet "and barley. And since we see that these can be separated "by a sieve, so in like manner water and oil are able to pass "through the pores of skin and of wood but air cannot, while "mercury can pass through the pores of gold but water, oil or "air cannot. Consequently the said fluids can be separated "(just as vegetable grains may be) from other different fluids "with which they may be mixed by means of a sieve of an "appropriate structure without any fermentation; for just as

"grains pass through a sieve uninjured, so oil and water can
"pass through the pores of skin or wood, intact, without any
"change. Wherefore it must be confessed that it follows by
"mechanical laws that the reason why fluids of the one kind
"do pass through and those of another kind do not is without
"doubt because the shapes of the molecules of the said fluids
"match and are fitted to the shapes of the minute pores
"through which they are able to pass while the particles of
"another fluid, since their shapes do not match, are ex-
"cluded."

And dwelling on the secretion of urine he concludes:

"Who then would wish to think that the particles of the
"blood are picked out, separated from the watery particles
"(of the urine) and placed in separate receptacles by some
"magnetic virtue or by some ferment, acting like a servant
"possessing eyes? Certainly unless we wish to lay hold of
"follies and wonders we are bound to confess that (in the
"kidneys) there exist two kinds of orifices after the manner
"of two sieves, namely, one a venous one, which by reason
"of its adjusted configuration receives the particles of blood
"only, not those of the watery urine, and another, the proper
"vessels of the kidneys, the shapes of which are fitted for
"absorbing the particles of water but not the particles of the
"blood."

With the history of the physiology of secretion I propose
to deal in a general way presently, and will therefore content
myself with thus much of Borelli's views. But I must say one
word about his views of the physiology of nerves, though to
these also I shall have to return later on.

The animal spirits of the older writers become in his hands
a nervous fluid, a fluid subtle and active but still a fluid
subject to the physical laws of fluid, which he calls *succus
nerveus*. He further distinguishes between a *succus nerveus
nutritivus* and a *succus nerveus spirituosus*. The former governs
the nutritive processes of the body, it is through these that
nerves exert what we now call a trophic action, the blood
supplying material, the nerves the vivifying and plastic force.

The *succus spirituosus* is concerned in the production of
movements and sensations, it is a fluid subject as we just now

said to physical laws. He develops his views as to the mechanical arrangements which determine its flow along the nerves, and in one place compares a nerve to a rod of elder-pith filled with fluid and so through the fluid capable of transmitting oscillations. And throughout he insists that the nervous fluid, the *succus nerveus*, is essentially a physical fluid. Such a fluid, says he, be it as spiritual, as subtle, and as active as you please, is always corporeal and is incapable of acting at a distance.

He also discussed in the same spirit the *succus spirituosus seminalis* (Auber, under his supervision, discovered in 1657 at Pisa the true structure of the testicle), the generation and nutrition of both plants and animals, and even the nature of several diseases.

When we pass in review the various instances of the firm, sharp, decided way in which Borelli laid hold, with his physical methods, of a whole series of problems, taken from nearly all parts of physiology, in dealing with which while we can now see how often he went wrong, we must also acknow-ledge how often he was right, how often he brilliantly hit the mark, two reflections force themselves upon us.

In the first place when we remember that Borelli's book was published some fifty years only after the appearance of Harvey's work, and that he appears to have been teaching publicly much that is contained in it very many years before it was published, we are impressed with the enormous progress in physiology during the interval, a progress due in the main to the development of the new physical mechanical mathematical philosophy.

In the second place, when we consider the effect which a perusal of Borelli's book has upon the reader now, we can easily understand how he was a founder of a great school which flourished long after him. He was so successful in his mechanical solutions of physiological problems that many coming after him readily rushed to the conclusion that all such problems could be solved by the same methods. And as is often the case, the less qualified, alike as regards mechanical as well as physiological knowledge and insight, to follow in Borelli's path were the men of succeeding times, the more loudly did they often proclaim the might of Borelli's method. Thus there came in the times after Borelli a school who, imitating and often mimicking Borelli, proposed to explain all physiological phenomena by the help of mathematical formulae and of hypotheses concerning forces and the shapes and sizes of particles, the iatro-mathematical or iatro-physical school, whom I shall frequently have occasion to mention in succeeding lectures.

LECTURE IV

MALPIGHI AND THE PHYSIOLOGY
OF GLANDS AND TISSUES

THE rapid development of mechanical and physical science
was not the only event taking place in the beginning of the
seventeenth century which profoundly influenced the progress
of physiology. The introduction of the microscope, though
acting in a different way, proved itself an aid of almost equal
importance to biological studies, though its effects did not
make themselves felt until more than half the century had
run its course.

The anatomists of the sixteenth century, and of the early
part of the seventeenth century, were content like their fore-
fathers to carry on their studies with what we now call the
naked eye, unassisted by any optical instruments. Hence their
statements as to the finer structure of the various organs and
parts of the body were necessarily vague and incomplete.
They could tease certain parts more or less completely into
strands of greater or less thickness and hence could speak of
fibres and of fibrous structure. They recognized skins and
membranes of various thickness. They were able to distinguish
what we call fatty or adipose tissue by means of its gross
features. And they could follow out the blood vessels and
later on the lymphatic vessels until these were lost to view
as minute channels. Beyond this, they were content to speak
of that part of the substance of an organ which could not be
split into fibres, and into which the minute vessels seemed to
disappear, as 'parenchyma,' using the word introduced in
ancient times by Erasistratus, but no longer attaching to the
word the original meaning of something poured out from the
veins. By parenchyma they simply meant the parts which
were not distinctly made up of fibres and which in most cases
at least were porous. Thus Harvey speaks of the blood which
flows along the pulmonary artery as being discharged into
the porous parenchyma of the lungs and gathered up thence
by the beginnings of the pulmonary veins. The histology, if
we may so use the word, of these older writers was of a simple
kind. Glisson, of whom I shall have to speak later on in other

connections, in the anatomical introduction to his treatise on
the liver, gives, in his usual formal didactic style, a sketch
of the current views as to the morphological constitution of
the animal body.

He divides the body into similar parts and organic parts,
the former being determined by the material of which they
are composed, the latter by the form which they assume. This
division comes obviously very near our ordinary division into
tissues and organs.

The similar parts or tissues may be again divided into the
sanguineous, or those which are richly provided with blood,
and the spermatic which are not, but he observes that the
differentia between these is not an exact one.

The spermatic tissues he divides again into the soft, such
as brain, the hard, such as bone, and the tensile; the last he
again divides into membranous tissues, such as the pia mater
and the peritoneum, fibrous tissues, such as the tendons and
ligaments as well as the fibres of muscle, of the heart and
possibly of the kidneys, and the tissues which are composed
of both fibres and membranes, such as the true skin, the
tissues of the intestines and others.

The sanguineous tissues are the fatty tissues and the
parenchymatous, the latter being either properly sanguineous,
such as the heart, lungs, kidney and liver, or phlegmatic, such
as the testicle, the pancreas and some other glands. He states
that the fleshy parts of muscles as distinguished from the
fibres of muscle are by some regarded as another variety of
the sanguineous tissues, but in his opinion are really parenchymatous.

Though, when Glisson wrote this, the new aids had already
come into use, and indeed he speaks of the advantages of
using optic tubes and microscopes in examining the pores of
the parenchymatous tissues, he himself had obviously had
but little if any recourse to these aids, and his exposition may
be taken as that of the views held before the microscope was
effectively used.

The invention of the microscope, that is of the compound
microscope (for the simple lens was occasionally used from
very early times), is a matter of some dispute. It has been

attributed to Fontana and also to Galileo, but the general opinion is that the first instrument was invented, some time before 1610, possibly in 1590, by the brothers Hans and Zacharias Janssen, of Middelburg in Holland; the one made by these is said to have been 1½ feet in length. Cornelius Drebbel, of Alkmaar in Holland, is however credited with having made at almost the same time an improved and really effective instrument; and to him the introduction of this new optical aid is mainly due.

It was not until many years after its invention that the microscope was seriously applied to anatomical studies. Francisco Stelluti is said to have been the first thus to use it at Rome in 1625, a year after the new invention had found its way to Italy; but the men who by its use opened up a new path in anatomy and started new ideas were four—Marcello Malpighi of Bologna, Anton van Leeuenhoek of Delft, Robert Hooke of London, and Johannes Swammerdam of Amsterdam. Of these by far the greatest from a physiological point of view was Malpighi.

Born at Crevalcore, close by Bologna, where his parents, well-to-do people, possessed a small farm, on the 10th of March, 1628, the year of the publication of Harvey's book, Marcello Malpighi entered in 1645 the University of Bologna as a student in philosophy. In this he made rapid progress, but in 1649 his studies were interrupted by the death, almost at the same time, of his father, his mother, and his father's mother. Full of affection as a boy, and he was no less so as a man, he was at first prostrated at the loss. Moreover as the eldest of a family of eight, three of whom next to him were girls, his hands were full in the settlement of the patrimony, settlement rendered all the more difficult by reason of a dispute concerning boundaries which had arisen between the Malpighi family and the family of Sbaraglia, the possessors of an adjoining property. This dispute was continued on until the end of Malpighi's days and in course of time widened from a mere quarrel about land into a bitter and sustained effort on the part of the Sbaraglia family to do harm in every possible way to Malpighi's fame and welfare. Hence though he returned to the University for a short time in the succeeding year, it was not until the year after, in 1651, that he definitely resumed his studies, and then with the view of entering upon the profession of medicine.

The Obscurantists, the Galenists were at that time still powerful in the University; but Bartolommeo Massari, Professor of Medicine, was full of the new learning. Not content with the formal duties of his Chair, he in 1650 gathered together at his own house some of the younger professors and older students, forming them into a club to which later on, the number of members becoming limited to nine, the number of the Muses, the name of the *Corus anatomicus* was given. Stimulated by Harvey's new views and by the discovery of the lacteals, the enthusiastic nine made their meetings the occasion not only for discussions but also for dissections on dead bodies, and experiments on living animals. Into their number the young Malpighi was soon admitted, and in what he learnt at their meetings he laid the foundations of his future work. Accurate and unwearied in study, bright in mind, quick to grasp each new thing, but withal mild, retiring and affectionate in disposition, he soon gained the love and esteem of his teacher, and so rapidly did he profit by what he was taught that in two years, in 1653, he became Doctor in Medicine and Philosophy.

As doctor he had a right to expect that he would be allowed to deliver a course of lectures; but not only as the pupil of Massari but also and perhaps by reason of what he was already shewing himself to be, he was in disfavour with the Obscurantists in power, and the right was for a time denied him. Meanwhile he drew closer the bonds which bound him to his teacher by marrying, in 1654, Francesca, Massari's sister, who, though she bore him no children, stood by his side until a few weeks before his death, a tender, cultivated helpmeet. The next year both were plunged in grief by Massari's sudden death; but in the year after that, in 1656, Malpighi, who meanwhile had been busying himself in medical practice, obtained at last a Chair, and was made a Professor of Medicine.

By that time however his already conspicuous ability had become known outside Bologna, and in the same year Ferdinand II, Grand Duke of Tuscany, always on the look-out to encourage and develop the powers of promising young men, and endeavouring with princely magnificence to make potent and famous the University of Pisa, created for him there a new special Chair of Theoretical Medicine, or as we might say, of the Institutes of Medicine, *i.e.* of Physiology. Malpighi, feeling acutely the opposition to himself and to his family in his native city, accepted the offer.

Here at Pisa he laboured for three years, enjoying and stimulated by the brilliant intellectual activity of the place, where every effort to extend the bounds of natural knowledge was encouraged by not only the approval but also the material aid of Ferdinand. He profited much by daily intercourse with the bright minds which he met there, more especially with Borelli, who had come to Pisa in the early part of the same year. The two became close friends, being perhaps drawn to each other by the contrasts of their characters. Borelli, twenty years older than Malpighi, self-asserting, confident, claiming as his own not only what he had done but at times what had been done by others, angry if his own merits were not fully acknowledged, impatient of the praises of others, bore himself, as we have said, in daily life with a taciturn coldness if not with a rough fretfulness, which kept many who admired his talents from looking upon him as a friend. Malpighi, kindly even to softness, ready to give his affections to those who seemed drawn to him, devoted wholly to those who had won his love, modest and retiring even to timidity, bold only in the interests of truth and right, never in his own, lived a life such as the sweet delicate outlines of his face bespoke, beloved for the sake of himself, even by those who were not competent to judge of his talents and his works. Two things the two had in common; each of them possessed a fragile frame buffeted by repeated ailments, each was moved to the depths of his being by a passion for the new learning. Each was able to learn from the other. Borelli could teach Malpighi the new mathematical physical learning of the school of Galileo, of which there does not seem to have been at this time any adequate exponent at Bologna, so that Malpighi came to Pisa with much yet to know. Malpighi on the other hand was able to lead Borelli into pastures of

anatomical inquiry as yet new and fresh to him, for, so far
as can be learnt, Borelli's mind was not, until he came to
Pisa, turned towards those biological problems which occupied
so much of his subsequent life. The work done by Borelli,
on which I dwelt in the last lecture, was begun, and indeed
much of it was at least hewn out in the rough, with Malpighi
at his side. Day by day, after their lectures were over, they
met at Borelli's house or elsewhere, either with other friends
present or without them, dissecting, experimenting and discussing. They even listened to each other's lectures, for there
is a story that at one of Malpighi's early lectures, the new
doctrines which he expounded so offended his audience, that
they one after the other withdrew, until at last Borelli was
left as the sole listener. Malpighi was ever ready to insist
upon the great help which he received from Borelli, and if
Borelli was less ready to acknowledge what he had gained
from his younger friend, this, in the judgment of posterity,
seems to have been at least not less, perhaps greater, possibly
much greater than the former. Much as Malpighi owed to
Borelli, great as was the guidance which in his early years
he had from him, he did not blindly adopt all Borelli's doctrines, and indeed as we shall see struck out new lines for
himself, being in many respects a wider thinker and a greater
man. This later divergence went far perhaps to bring about in
after years some estrangement between the two; but during
their common stay at Pisa, and for some time afterwards,
their friendship, though tried from time to time by Borelli's
behaviour, remained steadfast; whenever a new discovery or
a new idea came to Malpighi his first desire was to learn what
Borelli had to say about it.

Three years he thus spent at Pisa, teaching and learning,
busying himself among other things with experiments on the
blood more or less chemical, the results of which he recorded
after the fashion of the time in a Dialogue between a Galenist
and a surgeon of the new school. This however he did not
publish, and the manuscript was accidentally burnt years
after when his house took fire.

Meanwhile the domestic difficulties touching the paternal
estates at home increased rather than diminished; and prob-

ably in part in order to be on the spot but also for the reason stated by himself that the humid climate of Pisa, trying to many at the present day, was injuring his health, he asked permission of Ferdinand to resign his Chair and returned to his native city.

Here he resumed office as a Professor of Medicine, and, in spite of domestic troubles and anxieties, pursued his researches to such good effect that he was able in the next year, 1660, to announce privately to Borelli his discovery of the structure of the lung, an account of which was published in the year following. But his native city did not keep him long. In 1662, the chief or first Chair of Medicine in the University of Messina, then active, flourishing and ambitious, had become vacant, through the death of P. Castello, and the Senate, led to do so by the urgent advice of Borelli, who as we said in the last lecture had been professor there, offered, in April, the Chair to Malpighi, accompanying the offer with the promise of a handsome salary, as well as an adequate sum for the expenses of the journey. Malpighi for a while hesitated, distrusting his mental as well as his physical powers, but persuaded by Borelli, and influenced perhaps by dislike of the intrigues against him and his family going on in Bologna, finally accepted and after a brief stay at Naples on the way out entered upon his duties in the autumn of the same year.

Here for some four years, years fertile as we shall see in ideas, he remained, unwearied in labours of research, content with his position and with his work. Here he began a number of inquiries, some of which brought forth results ready almost at once to be made known, but others of which needed for their completion the toil of many years yet to come. Living close by the sea-shore he had ample opportunities for studying the anatomy of fishes and other creatures of the sea; and the simpler structures which he found in these opened up in his mind views as to the real nature of the like but more complex structures of man and the higher animals. It is perhaps not too much to say that during these four years there came to him many of the ideas to develop which was the work of his lifetime. His quiet undisturbed life in Messina was the germinal period of his career.

But Sicily was not his home, and was not to be his home. When, in 1666, the term of his appointment for four years had come to an end, the Senate of Messina pressed him, in so flattering a way, to continue in the Chair that he felt unable to refuse; but he asked and obtained leave to pay a flying visit to his native city. This he wished to do for one reason among others that he might give personal attention to the still troublous affairs of the family. He set out in the spring, staying on his journey for a few days at Rome, where he met and made friends with Stensen. The warm welcome with which he was received at Bologna was a token of the fame which his researches were already gaining for him. So great indeed had that fame become that his enemies could not withstand it, and his friends found themselves in a position to offer him the Chair of Medicine in his native city. This Malpighi accepted, and the Senate of Messina though much against their will set him free from the promise which he had made to them. He never returned to Sicily, but definitely took up once more a place in his old University. Here for a quarter of a century he remained, labouring not only in season but also out of season, for the feebleness of his body brought to him again and again times in which he ought to have folded his hands, but in which his active mind kept him still at work. Here he gave his lectures, here he went about healing the sick, and here all the time the best energies of his mind were being given to the task of penetrating the secrets of nature hidden in living bodies. He published the results of the inquiries which he had finished at Messina, he completed those which he had only begun there, and he carried on others wholly new. During the winter the duties of his Chair kept him closely confined to the city; but in the summer, when his lectures were over, it was his custom to retire to some quiet spot in the country near. Here, free from the interruptions incidental to a town life, he could give unbroken attention to his inquiries; the calm repose and the pure air of the fields gave renewed vigour to his feeble frame; and, in the loving company of his devoted wife, he spent golden days, observing, thinking and writing.

While he was yet at Messina the fame of his discoveries had reached the distant shores of England, and on his return to Bologna he received in 1667, forwarded to him from Messina, a letter from Oldenburg, the secretary to the newly established and almost feverishly active Royal Society of London, inviting him to a philosophic correspondence. That letter was the beginning of a long and close intercourse between the Italian philosopher and the English learned Society, one fruit of which was that the Royal Society had the honour of publishing and of bearing the expense of publication of the greater part of Malpighi's works, in fact with some slight exceptions of all the works which he produced after his return to Bologna.

Were I to attempt to do full justice to the memory of Malpighi I should have to go far beyond the limits of the subject of these lectures. He was the founder of, he opened up the path of inquiry in more than one branch of biological knowledge. He with the Englishman Nehemiah Grew laid the first sure foundations of vegetable morphology. While at Messina, walking one day in the garden of his friend and patron the Visconte Ruffo, snapping the branch of a chestnut tree which overhung and obstructed the path along which the two friends were walking his attention was arrested by the vascular bundles, projecting and hanging down from the broken end of the branch. This led him to study, and afterwards to write an immortal book on the Anatomy of Plants. The first sketch of this he sent to the Royal Society of London, which subsequently published the full work, and the day, December 7, 1671, on which it was presented and read before the Society happened to be the day on which Grew presented to the Society his printed book 'The Anatomy of Vegetables begun,' the order to print which had been given at a meeting of the Council of the Society in the previous May. The two inquirers struck upon the same ore, at the same time; and to both credit is due. But everyone who has read the two works by the two men must acknowledge that while that of the Englishman is a sound piece of honest, arduous labour, that of the Italian, no less sound, though perhaps less abounding in valuable detail, shines, more than does the other, with the light of genius, and is richer than the other in philosophic insight.

Malpighi may also be regarded as, almost in the same degree, the founder of that great and important branch of biological science which we call embryology. Long ago Aristotle had seen and studied the chick forming in the egg. More recently as we have said Fabricius had examined and described at some length the same mysterious events. Harvey in his later years had given his mind to the problem of the generation of animals. But none of these had gone very far. The first adequate description of the long series of changes by which, as they melt the one into the other, like dissolving views, the little white opaque spot in the egg is transformed into the feathered, living active bird, was given by Malpighi. And where he left it, so for the most part the matter remained until even the nineteenth century. For this reason we may speak of him as the founder of embryology.

He was also a zoologist, at least a comparative anatomist. Surrounded as he was in Italy, and even more so in Sicily, by cultivators of the silkworm, his correspondent Oldenburg, the secretary of the Royal Society, had in his letter invited him "to make the Society acquainted with any observations "made in Italy which he might think worthy of recounting, "and in particular observations on the silkworm and its "economy." Malpighi accordingly devoted himself to an exhaustive study of the silkworm in its various phases, examining not only its outward form but also the internal arrangement and the minute structure of all its viscera, leaving his name as Malpighian tubules on certain of them, and tracing out the whole history of the creature from the egg to the perfect insect. The results at which he arrived he embodied in a treatise presented in the form of a letter to the Royal Society, the first of his books published by that body.

This was his chief work in comparative anatomy, a model work of supreme excellence, but he also made many other valuable observations on various animals, vertebrate and invertebrate.

Malpighi was no mere professor, his time was not spent wholly in the laboratory and lecture room. He was actively engaged in healing the sick, he was as familiar with the phenomena of disease as with the phenomena of the healthy living being. He brought to bear on the former the same clear intellect which he turned towards the latter, seeking to find out the causes of the events which he witnessed. He was as busy in the post-mortem room as in the dissecting theatre, and his writings on the characters and causes of disease justify us in claiming for him the merit of having laid the foundations of scientific pathology.

But it is not of Malpighi as botanist, as embryologist, as naturalist, as pathologist, or as biologist, for from his varied studies he stands out as the man who first of all others laid firm hold of the fundamental principle of the essential identity of vegetable and animal life, that I have here to speak. He was all these, but he was also the first who calling into his aid the newly invented microscope, opened up the way for a true grasp of the minute structure of the tissues and organs of the animal body, and in so doing opened up also a new branch of physiology. He was the first histologist, and with the new histology came new ideas of the functions of many important parts of the body.

To Vesalius, to Fabricius and to Harvey, who looked upon the animal body as composed of a number of organs deftly joined together, the problems of physiology presented them-selves as a number of special problems of a mechanical nature, capable of being solved by mechanical methods, except in so far as, to use Vesalius' words, the qualities of the proper substance of each organ supplied the determining factor of its functions. The microscope revealed to Malpighi features of structure transcending mere mechanical notions. He saw that the tissues in their minuter structure were governed by laws of their own, by laws different from those which deter-mined the uses of machines; and thus there came to him the new conception of an animal morphology. And his views broadened as, while still regarding the study of man's structure as his first duty, he pushed his researches into the structure of many animals, vertebrate and invertebrate, and also of plants. All these studies more and more revealed to him general plans of structure and common laws of growth. As Harvey had been led to new views by studying the uses of animal organs viewed as machines, as Borelli had been led to other new views by regarding the phenomena of the animal body as subject to ordinary physical laws, so Malpighi was led to still other new views by this new thought that the material of the living body was subject to, and so its functions determined by, laws of structure proper to itself, laws which we now call morphological.

The first work which he published was that 'On the Lungs' (*De pulmonibus observationes anatomicae*) in 1661, in the form of two letters to his friend and master Borelli, describing the results of an inquiry which he carried out at Bologna immediately after his return from Pisa. Up to that time little or nothing was known of the real structure of the lung. It was spoken of as fleshy, and its substance, which Fabricius had compared to tow, was held to be a porous parenchyma, in which the minuter divisions of the blood vessels on the one hand and of the windpipe on the other were lost. It was into the spaces of this porous fleshy parenchyma, as we have said, that the blood of the pulmonary artery was supposed to be poured, thence to be gathered up by the beginnings of the pulmonary veins.

In these brief epistles Malpighi announced two discoveries of fundamental importance. In the first letter he described the vesicular nature of the lung and shewed how the divisions of the windpipe ended in the dilated air vesicles. He thus for the first time supplied an anatomical basis for the true conception of the respiratory process.

In the same epistle he describes the network of blood vessels, of arteries and veins (it may be worthy of note that Malpighi always speaks of the pulmonary artery and pulmonary veins, the old term of the artery-like vein and the vein-like artery having by this time become obsolete) winding over the air vesicles, but he could not as yet (he was so far working chiefly on the lungs of dogs) satisfy himself on the point whether or no the blood escaped from the minute arteries into empty spaces whence it found its way into the minute veins. A little later he turned his attention to the simpler lung of the frog, and in this he had the happiness, calling into his aid the microscope, to see that minute but definite channels, the channels which we now call capillaries,

joined the endings of the minute arteries to the beginnings of
the minute veins.

In his second epistle to Borelli, after describing, under the
heading 'I see with my own eyes a certain great thing,' the
appearances presented by the lung of the living frog extruded
after the laying open of the body, which organ he says "is
"nothing else than a sort of membranous bladder which at
"first sight seems to be sprinkled over with very little spots
"disposed in an orderly fashion like the skin of the dog-fish,
"commonly called Sagrino," he thus continues:

"Something still more wonderful than the above appear-
"ances which relate to mere structure and build is disclosed
"by microscopic observation. For, while the heart is still
"beating, two movements contrary in direction though ac-
"complished with difficulty are observed in the vessels so that
"the circulation of the blood is clearly laid bare; and indeed
"the same may be even more happily recognized in the
"mesentery and in other larger veins contained in the
"abdomen. And thus by this impulse the blood is showered
"down in minute streams through the arteries, after the
"fashion of a flood, into the several cells, one or other con-
"spicuous branch passing right through or leaving off there,
"and the blood, thus repeatedly divided, loses its red colour,
"and, carried round in a sinuous manner, is poured out on all
"sides until it approaches the walls, and the angles and the
"absorbing branches of the veins.

"The power of the eye could not be carried further in the
"opened living animal; hence I might have believed that the
"blood itself escaped into an empty space and was gathered
"up again by a gaping vessel and by the structure of the
"walls. But an objection to this view was afforded by the
"movement of the blood being tortuous and scattered in
"different directions and by its being united again in a deter-
"minate part. My doubt was changed into certainty by the
"dried lung of the frog which to a very marked extent had
"preserved the redness of the blood in very minute tracts
"(which were afterwards found to be vessels) where by the
"help of our more perfect glass there met the eye no longer
"scattered points resembling the skin which is called Sagrino,

"but vessels joined together in a ring-like fashion. And such
"is the wandering about of these vessels, as they proceed on
"this side from the vein and on the other side from the artery
"that the vessels no longer maintain a straight direction, but
"there appears a network made up of the continuations of the
"two vessels. This network not only occupies the whole area
"but extends to the walls, and is attached to the outgoing
"vessel, as I could more abundantly and yet with greater
"difficulty see in the oblong lung of the tortoise, which is
"equally membranous and transparent. Hence it was clear
"to the senses that the blood flowed away along tortuous
"vessels and was not poured into spaces, but was always
"contained within tubules, and that its dispersion is due to
"the multiple winding of the vessels. Nor is it a new thing in
"Nature to join to each other the terminal mouths of vessels,
"since the same obtains in the intestines and other parts;
"and, indeed, what seems more wonderful, she joins together
"by a conspicuous anastomosis the upper and lower termina-
"tions of veins as the most learned Falloppius has very well
"observed.

"In order, however, that you may more easily grasp what
"I have just stated, and follow it with your own eyes, ligature
"with a thread at the spot where it joins the heart the pro-
"truded and turgid lung of a frog whose body has been laid
"open, doing this while a copious supply of blood is flowing
"through the whole of it.

"This even when dried will preserve its vessels turgid with
"blood. And this you will see exceedingly well if you examine
"it with a microscope of a single lens against the horizontal
"sun. Or you may adopt another method of seeing these
"things. You will place on a transparent plate the lung,
"illuminated from below by the light of a lamp conducted
"through a tube and you will bring to bear upon it a micro-
"scope of two lenses. In this way the vessels distributed in
"a ring-like fashion will be disclosed to you. By the same
"arrangement of the instrument and the light you will observe
"the movement of the blood in the vessels lying in the field
"of view. And you will yourself be able, with different degrees
"of light which escape description by the pen, to devise other

"things. Concerning the movement of the blood, however,
"one thing presents itself as worthy of your speculation. The
"auricle and heart being ligatured and so all movement and
"impulse which might be conveyed from the heart to vessels
"still connected with it being removed, the blood still flows
"towards the heart along the veins and distends these by its
"movement and copious supply; and this lasts for several
"hours. At the end however, especially if it be exposed to the
"sun's rays, it is not the subject of the same continued move-
"ment but as it were of alternating impulses; the blood,
"moving to and fro, progresses and then recedes along the
"same way. And this takes place also even when the heart
"and auricle have been removed from the body.

"Turning therefore to the former problems demanding
"solution, it may, by analogy, and from the simplicity which
"Nature uses in all her works, be concluded from these results
"that that network which I once thought to be nervous in
"nature is really a vessel attached to the vesicles and sinuses
"carrying thither the mass of the blood or carrying the same
"away, and that although in the lungs of the more perfect
"animals a vessel seems sometimes to leave off and to gape
"in the middle of the network of rings, yet it is probable that,
"as in the cells of the frog and the tortoise, the vessel in
"question is prolonged further into very small vessels after
"the form of a network, although these on account of their
"exquisite fineness escape our senses."

This was the first observation of the capillaries. A few
years later, in 1668, that patient and accurate Dutch observer
Anton van Leeuwenhoek observed them in fishes and in
amphibia, and gave a fuller description of them. With the
clue thus given their presence was shewn or taken for granted
in all other structures, and it soon became acknowledged that
the circulation was a more complete mechanism even than
Harvey had supposed, that the blood flowed in wholly closed
channels from the heart through arteries, capillaries, and
veins back to the heart again. A sound view of the processes of nutrition thus became possible, and it was Malpighi
who first found the missing link in the chain of Harvey's
discovery.

In a little tract on the omentum, fat, and adipose ducts (*De omento, pinguedine, et adiposis ductibus*) published four years later, in 1665, in company with three other tracts of which I am about to speak, Malpighi records an observation which shews that he had hit upon another discovery touching the blood; but he failed to lay hold of the meaning of what he saw. Up to this time the redness of red blood had been supposed to be diffused over the whole fluid. Malpighi in describing the fat-cells, of which he found the fat of the omentum to be composed, states that, using the microscope, he fancied he saw small flat red cells in the mesenteric blood vessels of the hedgehog (his anatomical histological studies were carried out on almost all manner of animals). This is what he says:

"And I myself in the omentum of the hedgehog in a "blood vessel which ran from one collection of fat to another "opposite to it, saw globules of fat, of a definite outline, "reddish in colour. They presented a likeness to a chaplet "of red coral."

He mistook however the nature of what he saw. What evidently were blood corpuscles he thought to be fat cells passing from the fatty tissue into the current of the blood.

Meanwhile in thus seeing red blood corpuscles he had been anticipated by the great Dutch observer of minute structures, Johannes Swammerdam of Amsterdam. That great work of patient conscientious industry, *Biblia Naturae*, though not published until 1738, and then by Boerhaave, long after the author's death in 1680, contains the record of an observation made so early as 1658, seven years before the appearance of Malpighi's tract. Speaking of the blood of the frog he says:

"In the blood I perceived the serum in which floated an "immense number of rounded particles, possessing the shape "of as it were a flat oval but nevertheless wholly regular. "These particles seemed however to contain within themselves "the humour of other particles. When they were looked at "sideways they resembled transparent rods as it were and "many other figures, according, no doubt, to the different "ways in which they were rolled about in the serum of the "blood. I remarked besides that the colour of the objects

"was the paler the more highly they were magnified by means
"of the microscope."

After this we owe the first real accurate description of the
red corpuscles to Leeuwenhoek, who in 1674 in the *Philosophical Transactions* gave an account of the red blood
corpuscles in man, and in various papers carefully described
the blood corpuscles of different animals, shewing that while
circular in mammals they are oval in birds, frogs and fishes,
and proving that in all cases the redness of blood is due to
these red bodies.

The discovery of the capillaries and the first observation of
red blood corpuscles were achievements of no mean value;
but still more important perhaps than these were Malpighi's
labours, many and varied, on the structure of glands and
glandular organs.

Before I go on to speak of these, however, I must say a
few words concerning two little tracts which he published in
1665 during the last year of his stay at Messina, one on the
tongue (*De lingua exercitatio epistolica*), addressed to Borelli,
the other on the external organ of sense (*De externo tactus
organo exercitatio epistolica*), addressed to his Sicilian patron
Ruffo.

Fabricius had made known the distinction between dermis
and epidermis. The papillae of the tongue, being obvious
structures, had long of course been known; but the general
opinion was that they were organs secreting fluid and so
helping to keep the mouth moist; and the papillae of the skin
were wholly unknown.

Malpighi, beginning to work on the tongue but extending
his researches to the skin, discovered that lower layer of the
epidermis, the *rete mucosum*, which we more frequently now
call after him the Malpighian layer. The fact that the surface
of the tongue, when well dried, remained dry when kept extended out of the mouth, shewed him that the papillae could
not be structures whose purpose was to secrete fluid. He
traced the distribution of the nerves to them and concluded
that they were organs of taste. Having arrived at this view,
the thought occurred to him that the sense of touch might be
served by similar organs in the skin whose general structure

was so like that of the tongue. Knowing what to look for, he soon found that for which he was seeking. He was soon able to demonstrate the existence of papillae in the skin; and the fact that they were most abundant in those regions in which the sense of touch was most acute convinced him that he had in them discovered the organs of touch.

At the same time he published also in a letter to his old fellow-student at Bologna, Fracassato, a tract on the anatomy of the brain (*De cerebro exercitatio epistolica*). An important work on this subject had in 1664 been published by the Englishman Willis, whose name remains to us in the term 'circle of Willis.' That book, of which as well as of other labours of Willis I hope to speak in the proper place, contains much that is valuable, but it was as yet unknown to Malpighi, whose results were arrived at independently.

In this tract he shews with the help of the microscope that the white matter consists of round but flattened little fibres arranged in bundles whose course is difficult to follow, but which in any case form tracts connecting the surface of the brain with various regions of the spinal cord. He further shews that the grey matter is not confined to the surface of the brain where it is called cortex, but exists in scattered masses in the interior, disposed around the ventricles, and along the spinal cord. The nature of this grey matter he is in this tract unwilling to define exactly, but when he returned to the subject a little later he concluded that it was of a glandular nature.

In this he was misled by his success in investigating the glandular organs in general, the results of his inquiries into which were published in 1666, the year he left Messina, under the title of *De viscerum structura exercitatio anatomica*. To these researches we must now turn; and we may here fitly consider together with Malpighi's labours those of other men studying the same subject.

For this purpose it will be well to go back a little and pass in brief review what were the views held in the days before Harvey concerning the functions of the structures known as glands. Under the term gland, however, many of the older writers included also many other organs, such as the brain and the tongue, in fact almost all the viscera except the heart and alimentary canal; for their point of view was that of gross anatomy, not like ours that of physiology.

Of these glands attention was directed chiefly to three, the liver, the spleen, and the kidneys.

The functions of the kidney seemed in some respects fairly simple. Amply supplied with both veins and arteries, the substance of the kidney strained off, as Vesalius says, from the blood not only of the veins, but also of the arteries, some but not all of the serosity; and this gathered in the pelvis of the kidney as urine was conducted by the ureters to the bladder. The great difficulty was to understand how the substance of the kidney, dense and firm, most like the substance of the heart, says Vesalius, though destitute of fibres of its own, these being supplied only by its own arteries, veins and nerves, could effect this straining.

The functions of the liver too seemed to the men of those times to be fairly well understood by them; the view which they took was somewhat as follows. The vena portae carried to the liver nutritive material gathered up from the stomach and intestines, and by the excessive branching within the liver brought that material within the grasp of the soft parenchymatous hepatic substance. By help of this substance a concoction was effected, a sort of fermentation was carried on. In some such way as the crude juice of the grape is fermented into wine, with the separation on one hand of the heavier faex which settles to the bottom, and of the lighter foam which rises to the top, so the crude gross blood of the vena portae was purified by the hepatic substance into the purer blood which made its way by the vena cava to the heart, through the separation of two impurities. Of these the one, the lighter one, corresponding to the foam or yeast of fermenting must, escaped as yellow bile into the minute beginnings of the biliary duct, and was thence carried to the gall-bladder, from which it from time to time escaped into the duodenum. The other, the heavier muddy impurity, passed back as black bile, according to common belief Vesalius says, meaning thereby that he did not believe it, to the spleen, being carried thither by the veins.

About the spleen itself there was more divergence of opinion. Admitting that the black bile carried to it from the liver was by the substance of the spleen acted upon and altered in some way, authorities were not agreed as to what followed. Most were of opinion that black bile acted upon by the spleen was poured into the stomach, and so passing through the intestine was discharged with the faeces, having in the stomach, if not along the intestine, served some useful purpose. But while some maintained that there was a definite canal, leading from the spleen to the stomach, and indeed to the cardiac end of the stomach, along which this modified black bile passed, others supposed it to be carried by veins. Vesalius is very sarcastic over both one and the other of these as well as over other views of this matter, and scoffs at those who are anatomists by imagination and not by dissection. He obviously did not believe in any passage of material at all from the spleen to the stomach, whether by a special duct or by the veins. But the view was in one form or other very generally adopted; it served as the theoretic basis of medical practice, and is still preserved in the popular phrase of suffering from the spleen.

Other glandular bodies such as the pancreas, the salivary glands, the thymus and the thyroid, were known, as well as the lymphatic glands scattered over different parts of the body; little attention however was paid to these. Neither salivary glands nor pancreas were known to possess ducts; and all these varied bodies were regarded, if noticed at all, from the same point of view.

It will be remembered that before the establishment of Harvey's views blood was supposed to be carried by the veins to organs as well as from organs; and the ideas just sketched were in large measure based on the assumption of this double venous flow and ebb, to and fro. Hence, when the proof came that in each organ blood flowed to the organ through the arteries alone, through the organ from the arteries to the veins, and away from the organs along the veins always in one direction, all these old views demanded reconsideration.

We shall have to consider some of the glands again from the point of view of the uses of their juices, when we come to discuss the development of the more chemical side of physiology. Meanwhile we may treat them from the point of view of the mechanism of secretion and of the relation of this to the vascular system; this was the point of view of Malpighi, who entered very slightly, indeed hardly at all, into the discussion of chemical problems.

The first step was taken by John George Wirsung, who though a Bavarian by birth held in the middle of the seventeenth century the once so famous Chair of Anatomy at Padua. In a letter to Riolan dated 1643, he described the duct of the pancreas which he had discovered the year before. He speaks of its entrance into the duodenum close to the mouth of the biliary duct, and of its ramifications in the body of the pancreas. He says that he found it easy to pass a style through from the body of the gland into the duodenum, but difficult to pass the style from the duodenum into the duct, that the duct is present in man at all ages, that he found it in all the animals which he had examined, and that it could not be either an artery or a vein, since it never contained blood, but on the contrary was often filled with a nearly colourless fluid which like bile stained a silver style.

Wirsung's pupil John Maurice Hofmann claimed the discovery as his own, as one made by himself and laid hold of by his master; but there is no satisfactory evidence of this. Wirsung met some years afterwards with a tragic death, being shot as he was entering his house at night; the legend states that a quarrel about the discovery of the duct was the cause of the murder, but it seems to have been the result of some private grudge.

Wirsung never followed up his discovery of the pancreatic duct by any study of the function of glands; and the new fact remained, so far as he was concerned, barren.

The next step was taken by the Englishman Thomas Wharton, who, born in 1614, seems to have carried out his medical studies exclusively in London, where he subsequently practised as a physician, being a great friend and ally of Glisson. In 1656 he published under the title of *Adenographia*, an exhaustive treatise on glands, the outcome of the anatomical lectures which he had given at the College of Physicians in 1652. In this he describes the anatomy, *i.e.* the external form and naked eye structure (for he does not seem to have used the microscope), and especially the arrangement of nerves, blood vessels and lymphatics, of all those organs in the body which he called glands, including in that term the brain and tongue. In the course of his description he gives an account of the discovery which he had made of the duct of the submaxillary gland, the duct which has since borne his name. He insists that by this duct real saliva, not mere phlegm or mucus, is discharged into the mouth. He also develops a theory of the use of glands, both of those having a duct and of those having none, which is worth noticing as illustrating some of the views of the period. While not denying that the blood brought to the gland by the arteries supplied the gland with material, and, in the case of a gland with a duct, furnished a part at least of the juice, he attached much greater importance to the nerves, and to the *succus nerveus*, which they carried; he like Borelli and others adopts this new term for the old animal spirits. He points out that most glands are richly provided with nerves, and argues that these nerves play one or other or both of two parts. They either give up something by the removal of which the succus nerveus is purified, the too great humidity of the nerves being thus lessened, the matter so transferred from the nerves to the gland leaving the gland by its duct, or in the absence of a duct, by the veins or lymphatics; or they take something from the gland by which means the succus nerveus is fortified.

It is obvious that Wharton was far from grasping the true meaning of his remarkable discovery.

The next step was taken by Nicolas Stensen, in Latin, Nicolaus Steno, the Dane of whom I have already spoken, and who in 1661 discovered and in the following year described the duct of the parotid gland, since called by his name.

Before speaking of this part of Stensen's work, I should like to say a few words about the life of this remarkable man.

Born at Copenhagen on January 10, 1638, his father being a court jeweller, zealous beyond measure in Lutheran doctrines, he studied medical subjects first in his native city under Bartholin, who assisted largely in the development of

the knowledge of the lymphatics then taking place, subsequently at Leyden under Sylvius, of whom I shall later on
have to speak, and later on under Blasius at Amsterdam. It
was while at work dissecting in the house of the latter that
he made his discovery of the duct.

His studies however had not been narrowly medical; as
shewn by his work on muscle of which we spoke, he had laid
a firm hold on the new mathematical and physical learning.

After publishing in 1662, while as yet a young man of
twenty-four years, his *Observationes Anatomicae* relating his
discovery of the parotid duct, he travelled much in Germany,
France, and other countries, mixing with learned men, learning not a little and also teaching not a little wherever he went.
It is said that at Paris he attracted the attention of the great
Bossuet, who desired to convert him to the Catholic religion,
but Stensen told him that he was far too busily occupied with
science to be able to attend to such matters. At one of his
visits to Paris he was invited to deliver at a meeting of learned
men held in the house of Thévenot, a discourse on the Anatomy
of the Brain. In this discourse, published in 1669, which we
have already quoted, he criticizes in a fearless and severe
manner, from the point of view of the exact anatomist and
physiologist, the fanciful and popular views put forth by
Descartes.

After a while, in 1666, he came to Italy, staying some time
in Padua, and then going on to Pisa. Here he attracted so
much attention that Ferdinand II invited him to Florence to
be Court Physician, a post in which Cosimo III on his succession confirmed him, entrusting him at the same time with
the education of his children.

While thus engaged, still working at physiology, he turned
his versatile mind to other problems as well, to those of
comparative anatomy, and especially to those of the infant,
indeed hardly as yet born, science of geology. His work *De
solido intra solidum* is thought by geologists to be a brilliant
effort towards the beginning of their science.

In 1672 he returned for a while to his native city of Copenhagen, but within two years he was back again at Florence;
and then there came to him, while as yet a young man of

some thirty-six summers, a sudden and profound change in his life.

In his early days he had heard much, too much perhaps, of the doctrines of Luther. Probably he had been repelled by the austere devotion which ruled the paternal roof. And, as his answer to Bossuet shews, his university life and studies, his intercourse with the active intellects of many lands, and his passion for inquiry into natural knowledge had freed him from passive obedience to dogma. He doubtless, as did many others of his time, looked upon himself as one of the enlightened, as one raised above the barren theological questions which were moving the minds of lesser men.

One day however visiting at Florence the pharmacy attached to Santa Maria Novello (the same pharmacy at which to-day you may buy orris root and other preparations), in order to purchase some drug, the holy brother who sold him the medicine for the body dropped some words about the remedies for the soul. The stray arrow entered between the joints of the harness. New thoughts were stirred up in the mind of the man of science and of the world; and within a year, to the astonishment of his friends, and to the dismay of all friends of the new learning, he forsook all his old studies, gave up all inquiry into the works of nature, and by taking orders solemnly devoted himself henceforward to the works of God and religion.

A convert of such powers and of such a fame could not but be warmly received by the Church; and in 1677, receiving the titular honour of Bishop of Titiopolis in Greece, he was sent as Vicar Apostolic to the northern countries of Europe in the hope that he might win back to the true faith many of the erring ones in the land in which he had been born and bred.

Led apparently by the thought that he might turn the old weapons which he had wielded so well to the use of his new purposes, he began once more to teach anatomy in his native city of Copenhagen, the strange position of a Catholic Bishop professing a mundane subject in a heretic university being accepted by the authorities, and approved by the Church. But the position was false as well as strange; the changed voice no longer as of old spoke with authority and power; the zeal for knowledge which had in old days charmed men as they listened to him, no longer made itself felt; and zeal for good, however fervent, could not take its place. Stensen soon saw that it was false; he gave up wholly all such attempts to work his old life into his new calling. Resigning his chair he henceforward devoted himself to the more usual duties of a priest. For nine years he lived in Germany, first at Hanover and then at Schwerin, a life of severe self-denial, labouring constantly for the welfare of the poor, with no thought but that of winning souls for the Church. The privations which he laid upon himself, and the toils which he underwent for others, were too much for the body, which had once filled so much of his thoughts, and which he now held as a thing of nought. He wore himself to death; and in 1686 at the relatively early age of forty-eight passed away. The brilliant achievements of his early days and the sanctity of his later life made his name in different ways precious at Florence; and at the command of the Duke of Tuscany the emaciated corpse of one who had been at once an apostle of science and a martyr to the calls of religion was brought back to Florence and buried with public honours in the city fitted perhaps above all others to receive it, as being, like the dead one, at once famous for learning and zealous for the Church.

Stensen gives a graphic description of his discovery of the parotid duct. He relates how, while he was residing with and studying under Blasius, one morning, when he was engaged in dissecting the head of a sheep and examining the parotid gland, the style which he was using, inserted by chance it would seem into an opening in the duct, slipped easily down and struck with a sharp clink against the teeth; he recognized that he had discovered the duct of the gland. Wharton as we have seen had just before discovered the submaxillary duct; but the two men made very different uses of their two discoveries. Wharton blundered, led away by current ideas of the nerves and their animal spirits. Stensen, who had learnt from his master Sylvius of Leyden the distinction between conglomerate glands, such as the salivary glands and the pancreas, and conglobate glands, such as the lymphatics, laid hold of the idea that the former were secretory glands and hence must all have ducts. He soon found the duct of the sublingual gland, as well also as those of the small buccal glands, and cleared up the problem of the secretion of tears by the lachrymal gland, concerning which in spite of the lead given by older anatomists there was as yet much confusion. Further, so far as he was able, seeing that he appears to have used the simple lens chiefly and the microscope very little if at all, and that he had as yet no knowledge of the capillaries, he formed a conception of the process of secretion which went very near to the truth and served as a useful basis for further inquiry.

He recognized that the material for the production of saliva or of any other secretion of a secreting gland is brought by the blood of the arteries and is given up in the substance of the gland to the beginnings of the duct, as the blood is passing from the arteries to the veins by which it leaves the gland. He seems to have wanted only a knowledge of the minute microscopic structure of the gland, and of the relation of the capillaries to the secreting vesicles; had he possessed these he might have given an account of the process such as would be accepted even at the present day. As it is, his views stand in bright contrast to those of Wharton. Nerves, he says, serve only for movement or for sensation, and the nerves of a gland are of use for these purposes only. He speculates how the action of the nerves by inducing movement can affect the flow of saliva, and throws out the idea that it may be by bringing about constriction of the veins, since this by opposing the flow of blood would throw more material into the beginnings of the duct.

He is very clear as to the essential difference in nature between the conglomerate (secreting) glands provided with ducts and the conglobate (lymphatic) ductless glands, and points out that lymph flows only from the former, whereas it flows to and through the latter on its way to the venous system.

In yet another organ another discovery, an important aid to the doctrine of secretion, was made about this time.

In the year 1662 a pupil of Borelli's, one Laurentio Bellini, a Florentine of good family, whether or no related to the great

Venetian painters I cannot tell, published a little tract *De structura renum*. He was then a mere youth of nineteen years. The Duke of Tuscany had sent to Borelli a deer to be used for anatomical purposes, and Bellini, under Borelli's guidance, carefully examined the kidneys. He then saw what no one had seen before, that the substance of the kidney was composed of minute tubules, urinary canaliculi, radiating from the pelvis towards the surface. Eustachius had seen something of these, but he described them as 'fuscous sulci'; it was Bellini who really grasped their nature, and these straight tubuli uriniferi (for he did not distinguish between the twisted and the straight tubules) have since been known by his name. He described the tubules as opening into the pelvis of the kidney and, guided by the mind of his master Borelli, expounded a physical theory of the secretion of urine. The minute arteries, he says, discharge their contents into spaces in the parenchyma of the kidney, whence the aqueous serosity of the blood passes into the beginnings of the urinary canaliculi, while the rest of the blood finds its way out by the veins. The selection of the one path and of the other is determined by the size and configuration of the particles; those of the aqueous serosity fit into the canals of the canaliculi, those of the rest of the blood do not. We see here a typical instance of the mechanical theories of physiological events of which the master Borelli was so prolific.

For a while Professor of Anatomy at Pisa, later on Bellini became physician to Cosimo III at Florence. He wrote several books and achieved fame and fortune; but this discovery of the urinary tubules, made in his teens, was his chief, perhaps we may say his only valuable, contribution to physiology, and in this the hand with which he wrought was the hand of Borelli.

Lastly it must not be forgotten that in 1654 Glisson, to whom I have already referred, and of whom I shall have to speak more fully in a subsequent Lecture, published his work on the Liver. In that work he gave a very careful description of the anatomy of that organ, which though set forth in somewhat cumbrous, academic fashion, made a valuable contribution to our knowledge, especially perhaps in all that relates to the distribution of the vessels. We at the present day call these researches to mind when we speak of Glisson's capsule, a structure which he was the first accurately to describe. This is what he says: "This structure was wholly unknown to the "ancients and therefore has hitherto been without a name. I "was the first (unless I am mistaken) to discover it, which "I did twelve years ago when, at the mandate of the College "of Physicians of London, I delivered a course of public "lectures, and in preparation of that course removed the "parenchyma from the livers of a large number of animals." And he describes his method of tediously scraping away the parenchyma. So far however as the intimate structure of the secreting substance of the liver is concerned he left much untouched, much indeed that he could not touch, seeing that he made apparently no use of the microscope. He admits that the parenchyma of the liver is the principal part since all other structures seem simply subservient to it, and speaks of it as exercising a straining action, of serving the purposes of a filter; but Vesalius had done this long before him. It strains off on the one hand the bile, and on the other hand the pure blood; and the filtration or separation of the two humours takes place, he says, in the following way: "It is very probable "that parts or particles of which the parenchyma is composed "are of different natures so as to be allied on the one hand "to one of the humours to be secreted (the bile), and on the "other hand to the other humour (the pure blood). Whence "it comes about that those humours suit themselves to those "parts with which they have the greatest likeness and "affinity. And that is the beginning of the secretion of them. "The particles for instance which have the greatest affinity "to the bile humour attract this to themselves, and then pass "it on to the first beginnings of the biliary duct. In like "manner those particles whose business lies especially with "the pure blood attract this to themselves, and then carry it "to the capillary roots of the *vena cava*."

Hence when during his stay at Messina Malpighi was studying the structure of the viscera, the results of which study he did not however publish until his return to Bologna in 1666, he had before him the striking new discoveries of which I have just spoken, namely the discovery of the pancreatic duct in 1642 by Wirsung, of the submaxillary duct in 1652–6 by Wharton, of the parotid and other ducts in 1661 by Stensen, and of the structure of the kidney in 1662 by Bellini. He was also acquainted with the distinction between conglomerate and conglobate glands made by Sylvius, as well as with the researches of Glisson on the liver and of Stensen on glands in general.

What use did he make of these, and how much further did he carry us?

Malpighi's book on the viscera contains an account of the study of four organs, the spleen, the kidney, the liver, and the cortex of the brain.

We may say at once that in his tract on the cerebral cortex he shewed that he was not infallible; carried too far by the enthusiasm for glandular structures which the works just mentioned had excited, he maintained that the cortex of the brain was also glandular; he described the superficial grey matter as glands hanging on to the strands of the white fibres like the fruit of the date palm.

In his tract on the liver he modestly says that Glisson had left him little to say, and yet the little which he did say was of prime importance. He for the first time shewed that the liver was constructed after the fashion of a conglomerate secreting gland, that its substance was arranged in small masses essentially like those of which a conglomerate gland such as the pancreas was made up; to these he gave the name of acini. Henceforward the mystery which had for so long hung over the liver was cleared away; the liver secreted bile after the same fashion that the parotid and submaxillary glands secreted saliva.

This is what he says:

"Since in the higher, more perfect, red-blooded animals, the "simplicity of their structure is wont to be involved by many "obscurities, it is necessary that we should approach the "subject by the observation of the lower, imperfect animals." He accordingly studies in the snail the organ "which by its "position and the connection of its vessels obviously fulfils "the nature and function of a liver." This he finds "to be

"divided into a number of lobules, possessing not so much a
"spherical as a conical outline. Nor is Nature content to have
"made use of such a division merely; but, in a most liberal
"manner, has established a further division into very small
"parts, visible only by the aid of the microscope. For each of
"the lobules just described is made up of small rounded
"bodies, like berries (acini) crowded together after the fashion
"of a bunch of grapes, and connected with the whole lobule
"by means of vessels."

He traces out a similar structure in other animals, in fishes,
reptiles, mammals, and finally in man, pointing out that these
structural features had been dimly seen by others, as by
Glisson, who, most accurate observer though he was, was so
carried away by his preconceived idea of the continuity of
the parenchyma of the liver, as to refuse to see what was
clearly before his eyes. And he thus sums up:

"In constructing the liver the following seems to be the
"constant method of Nature. The vessels in the liver are
"distributed in branches carried hither and thither in the
"common sheath observed by Glisson, in a manner I say
"similar to that which we see in the lung. Around the ends
"of each of the vessels, even the slender ones, are attached
"lobules maintaining for the most part a conical outline,
"not unlike that arising from the division of parts already
"described as existing in the lungs; and we may observe a
"similar arrangement in the pancreas and other conglomerate
"glands.

"These lobules are clothed with an investing membrane
"of their own, and are joined together by membranous ties
"carried across from one to the other, so that only very small
"intermediate spaces or clefts appear between the sides of
"the lobules which are so adapted to each other that no
"interruption between them either great or small arises, the
"size, position and adaptation of the cones being changed as
"required. We have shewn the same thing more clearly in
"the lungs. It is to be observed, however, that the outline
"of the lobules is not the same in all animals, but varies
"within very wide limits.

*   *   *   *   *   *   *

"The glandular acini of which each lobule is composed,
"since they have a special circumscription, possess an outline
"of their own, which is for the most part hexagonal or poly-
"gonal. Hence they necessarily are joined to each other
"by special membranous ties in addition to the vascular
"branches; and certain interstices occur between them which
"are quite conspicuous in fishes and other lower animals, but
"are obscure in the higher animals.

"To each of these lobules, even to the very small ones, as
"may actually be observed or inferred from a variety of facts,
"are carried numerous branches of vessels. For the divisions
"of the vena cava, of the vena portae, and of the bile-duct
"ramify continuously throughout the whole mass of the liver,
"as Glisson, in that work of his on the liver which cannot be
"too highly praised, has very clearly shewn. In the lobules
"which constitute the outside surface of the liver, the blood
"vessel, spreading out from a centre, ramifies in all directions
"over the whole periphery, sending forth bifurcating branches
"by which the whole lobule is irrigated. And the same can
"(not) be doubted concerning the deeper parts. For although
"the actual eye of sense cannot, especially in the higher
"animals, reach the extreme ends of the vessels which open
"on to the glandular acini, yet we may follow them ade-
"quately with the eye of reason. For the whole mass of the
"liver is composed of these two factors, namely, the glandular
"acini, and the different terminations of the vessels. Where-
"fore in order that some common result may issue from this,
"some intercourse between the glandular elements and the
"vessels must necessarily take place.

"Moreover, in the liver Nature follows this rule that the
"branches of the vena portae play the part of arteries, as is
"indicated by the complexity of their coats; and so closely
"is the vena portae associated and connected with the bile-
"duct that the small divisions of both of them are closely
"wrapped together in the same sheath."

He concludes that both observation and reason shew that
the liver is to be regarded as a conglomerate gland, such as is
the pancreas. And "since it is a feature of conglomerate
"glands that they possess an excretory vessel of their own,"

as Sylvius and Steno have shewn, "since this is the rule of "nature in the parotid, in the pancreas, in the salivary glands, "the sweat glands, the lachrymal glands and others, since in "these dispersed through their proper substance there may be "seen a special vessel distinct from the other ordinary vessels, "such as veins, arteries and nerves, a similar structure must "be looked for in the liver." He infers that the bile-duct is the proper excretory duct of the liver.

He had to contend against a heresy recently put forth that the bile was secreted, not in the liver itself but in the gall-bladder by means of the blood vessels and membranes of that organ, and that it was carried thence to the liver to aid in the process of sanguification. Against such a view all the above anatomical results afforded irresistible arguments; but he clenched these by a vivisectional experiment. Laying open a kitten, he tied the common bile-duct close to its entrance into the duodenum, and by a median incision emptied the gall-bladder. In a short time the common duct and the bile-duct were filled with bile. He then put a ligature round the neck of the gall-bladder; the common duct and the bile-duct were still full of bile, and when with his finger he tried to press back their contents towards the liver, they returned with force when the finger was removed.

He thus concludes:

"Among various questions which arise out of the discoveries "which have been described, two stand out prominent. By "what mechanism is the bile separated in the glandular acini "of the liver, and what is the use of bile in the economy? "The illustrious Pecquet has made many deductions from the "principles of mechanics concerning the former; since, how-"ever, the structure of the acinus is so minute that it cannot "be laid bare by even the very best microscope, we can only "have recourse to hypotheses and to the working of similar "mechanisms in attempting to explain this." And such a labour he does not propose to take up.

As to the use of the bile he can only say "that it is probable "that after the food has been triturated (in the stomach) "juices of a different nature are poured upon it from the "glands of the liver and from the pancreas, for a purpose not "unlike that which appears in the cooking of food when out "of sweet, sour, and salt things mixed together, a new com- "position and a new taste are developed. Let the wide industry "of others carry matters further, I am contented to have "described the simple and rude structure of the liver."

The description itself, however, was neither simple nor rude. It brought clear light to what before was wholly dark or, at least, most obscure; and where Malpighi left the matter, there it remained, with little change, until the nineteenth century.

In his tract on the kidney he went far beyond Bellini. He shewed that in man at least the kidney really consisted of several kidneys, and that the several constituent kidneys might be distinguished as masses of Bellini's tubules arranged in the form of pyramids, the pyramids since known as the pyramids of Malpighi. He shewed how in each pyramid Bellini's tubules ended in orifices at the summit of the papilla which formed the apex of the pyramid, and further how in the cortex of the kidney the tubules were not straight as Bellini had described them, but curiously and irregularly twisted. Lastly he pointed out how many at least of these tubules began as inflated swellings or capsules, "round like the eggs of fishes," and how these capsules contained a knot of blood vessels, and so hung on to the small arteries as "apples hang on to the branches of a tree." And he stated his conviction that these capsules, which have ever since borne his name, must play an important part in the secretion of urine.

Thus in 1666 Malpighi had arrived at a clear conception of the structure of the kidney. And the world had long to wait for any further large addition to our knowledge on this score. It is true that we owe a minuter knowledge of the distribution of the renal blood vessels to the skilled injections of Ruysch, who, born in 1638 and called to the Chair of Anatomy at Amsterdam while Malpighi was at Messina, lived a life prolific in work far on in the next century, until 1731, work which was partly, and so far wrongly, directed towards undoing what Malpighi had done, making the blood vessels the agents instead of the aids of secretion. It is also true that Antoine Ferrein, Professor at Montpellier and at Paris, made, nearly a century later, in 1749, in company with many errors, and these very great ones, a slight contribution to our knowledge when he described the rays of straight tubules shooting up into the cortex, since known as the pyramids of Ferrein. Putting aside however these two things, we may almost say that our knowledge of the kidney remained where Malpighi left it, until in the generation which has just passed away Bowman took up the subject again.

Lastly, in his tract on the spleen, that organ to which in the past so much honour had been paid, to which had been attributed so many and such varied and important duties, Malpighi brought into a region thick with the mists and clouds of indistinct theories and speculation the dry light of exact inquiry; and the mists and clouds forthwith dispersed.

He gave a careful description of its structure, of its capsule, trabeculae and pulp, and of its blood vessels and nerves. The trabeculae he at first suspected to be nervous in character, but he soon recognized that in many animals they were muscular or at least contractile. "The fibres" (*i.e.* the trabeculae), he says, "of the spleen are not, as I once thought, nervous but "fleshy, so that by means of the external fleshy capsule and "the fibres carried transversely from it is formed a remarkable "muscle compressing the chambers of the spleen, in structure "and fashion not unlike what is seen in the larger auricles of "the heart." He thus shewed that the spleen was not a gland, either conglomerate or conglobate, but a contractile vascular organ such as we now recognize it to be. But he also recognized the possibility of changes of a peculiar nature taking place in the spleen pulp filling up the chambers just alluded to, all the more so since he was the first to observe small white bodies, not unlike glands, attached to the blood vessels, bodies which have ever since borne the name of Malpighian corpuscles. He also called attention to the remarkable reticular sheath which accompanies and wraps round the arteries as these plunge into the body of the organ.

All these several fundamental discoveries were made before he left Messina to take up his abode in his native city. During his long stay in Bologna he continued to labour at anatomical problems of physiological interest, and wrote important treatises, such as those on the uterus, on hairs, horns, bone, on the polypus of the heart, and especially one on the lymphatic glands published by the Royal Society in 1689 (*De structura glandularum conglobatarum, consimiliumque partium*); yet none of these made known results at all equal in importance to those on which we have just dwelt. During this time his intellectual strength was chiefly spent on researches not distinctly physiological, such as those on the anatomy of plants, on the formation of the chick, on the natural history of the silkworm, and others.

The years slipped away without any striking event breaking the even tenor of his way. His winters he spent in the city busy with his professorial and professional duties; his summers, as we have seen, were periods of repose and yet of labour in his summer retreat. In 1662 he bought a villa and small estate at Corticella in the neighbourhood of the city, and the possession of a country house of his own led him, as years grew upon him, more and more into rural retirement. In 1684 a great misfortune befell him. His house in Bologna caught fire, his microscopes were ruined and many of his precious manuscripts were burnt. The loss of his furniture and suchlike things he laughed at; but the destruction of his papers filled him with grief. Yet he did not despair, he persevered in labours of inquiry. The old family feud continued to molest him up to nearly his last days. In 1689, when he and his wife, both now advanced in years and feeble in health, were residing almost alone, or at most with the scantiest attendance, in their country villa, some of the Sbaraglia party thought it no shame to dress themselves up in grotesque costumes and make a burlesque attack upon the dwelling. Not content with frightening the infirm old man and his invalid wife, they attempted to injure his property and even to destroy his papers. Happily they were obliged to desist; but the incident illustrates some of the difficulties amid which Malpighi carried on his remarkable labours. With a name honoured throughout the world, surrounded by loving friends at home, stimulated and encouraged by the letters of other friends at a distance, especially perhaps by those of Bellini, having himself a character which would wish to be at peace with all men, his long life was throughout from time to time embittered by ignoble attacks taking origin from a paltry domestic dispute.

In 1691 Pope Innocent XII, soon after he ascended the papal throne, sent to Malpighi, whose worth he had learnt to value during the time in which as Antonio Pignatelli he had resided in Bologna, an invitation to come to Rome and be his physician. Malpighi at first refused; he was unwilling to leave his beloved city, his friends, his studies, and the country seat of which he had become so fond, and to take up his abode, now an old man near his end, in a strange city. But the Pope would not take a refusal, and in the end Malpighi, though unwillingly, accepted the invitation.

He left Bologna amid demonstrations of affection, esteem and regret, he was received at Rome with every possible manifestation of respect. And here for a while he continued the labours of his life. But not for long. Soon after his arrival at Rome he began to lose colour and flesh and to look ill. In July 1694 he had a slight apoplectic attack. From this however he soon recovered; but during his convalescence, which he spent chiefly in preparing for publication the writings which, under the care of the Royal Society, saw the light as his posthumous works, a heavy blow fell upon him— the death of his beloved wife who had stood by his side for so many years.

On the 28th of November a second stroke of apoplexy came upon him, this time heavy and fatal, and on the following day he passed away. At the post-mortem examination a very large effusion of blood was found in the right ventricle of his brain. By an irony of fate the right kidney of him, who had done so much to clear up the mysteries of renal structure, was found to be marked with old-standing disease; it was largely dilated, and indeed he had for most of his life suffered from renal calculi.

It may be truly said of Malpighi that whatever part of natural knowledge he touched he left his mark; he found paths crooked and he left them straight, he found darkness and he left light. Moreover in everything which he did there is the note of the modern man. When we read Harvey we cannot but feel that in spite of all which he did, he in a way belonged to the ancients; while he was destroying Galen's doctrines he was wearing Galen's clothes, and speaking with Galen's voice. When we pass to Malpighi we seem to be entering into the ways and thoughts of to-day. Doubtless Malpighi was reaping what Harvey had sown; doubtless he was also reaping what Galileo had sown; doubtless also the microscope gave him a tool which none before him had possessed. It was just the putting these three things together which parts him from the old times, and makes him the beginning of the new.

All the deeper problems of physiology turn on the mutual action of the tissues and the blood, as the stream of the latter sweeps among the elements of the former. Harvey shewed that the blood did sweep through the tissues, Malpighi shewed what the tissues were and how the blood swept through them. And thus the way was opened for those inquiries into the ways in which the blood acts on the tissue and the tissue acts on the blood, inquiries the results of which are the pride of modern times and the hope of times to come.

LECTURE V

VAN HELMONT AND THE RISE OF CHEMICAL PHYSIOLOGY

IN the work of the physiologist of to-day the teachings of chemistry are held, and rightly held, in high esteem. Though many problems in physiology may still be regarded, and, it may be, will always have to be regarded as purely physiological problems, as problems to be solved in their own way and by no other means, yet a preponderating number, perhaps also an increasing number of the problems on which the physiologist is to-day engaged, are at bottom chemical or physical problems, problems to be solved by the application of chemical or physical methods to the phenomena of living beings.

In a previous lecture I spoke of the influence on the progress of physiology exerted by the new physical learning which came into power in the early years of the seventeenth century; it was then that physics and physiology touched hands. I now propose to speak of the way in which chemistry came to the aid of those who were inquiring into the problems of life, and thus gave rise to the chemical physiology which we know to-day.

The physiology of Vesalius and his school consisted as we have seen of deductions from the data of anatomical arrangements confirmed or corrected by experiments on living animals. From time to time Vesalius made use of the growing mechanical knowledge of his age, and we trace here and there the influence of the as yet imperfect physical conceptions then dominant. But of chemistry as we now know it there is hardly a word. If you take up a text-book of modern physiology you will find page after page occupied with chemical matters. In some text-books digestion and its consequences take up so large a space as to suggest to the reader that the stomach is the larger part of man. It is not so with the writings of Vesalius. In that chapter in the *Fabrica* of which I have spoken as his compendium of experimental physiology, the whole of digestion and nutrition is dismissed in almost a single sentence. "Though there is no difficulty in examining

"living dogs at different times after they have been fed with
"the view of investigating the functions of the alimentary
"canal, yet we learn little more by vivisection than we do by
"the study of the dead body, as regards the function of the
"liver, spleen, kidney, or bladder. It may perhaps please one
"to excise the spleen, as I have done, the animal living many
"days afterwards."

There is, so far as I know, not a single reference in any
of Vesalius' writings to that study of the intimate nature of
things which under the name of chemistry, or rather of
alchemy, was beginning to stir men's minds and which was
pushing its way into the art of medicine. The great anatomist
would no doubt have made use of his bitterest sarcasms had
someone assured him that the fantastic school which was busy
with occult secrets and had hopes of turning dross into gold,
would one day join hands in the investigation of the problems
of life with the exact and clear anatomy so dear to him.

Nor did Harvey any more than Vesalius pay heed to
chemical learning. His book on the heart contains no more
references to this than do the writings of Vesalius, and even
his work on generation expounds only the chemistry of the
ancients.

During the sixteenth century, however, and still more in the
seventeenth century there grew up side by side, but as yet
apart from the physiology on which we have so far dwelt, a
knowledge having an origin quite separate from anatomy, and
indeed at first quite separate from the study of living things,
a knowledge of which subsequently every physiologist had to
make use. With this knowledge the men of the seventeenth
century of whom we have spoken, Borelli, Malpighi and others,
were not unacquainted; but as a rule the share which it had
in the guidance of their thoughts was a small one. To Borelli,
the spirit of inquiry as yet reigning in chemistry was so
different from that of the school of Galileo that though some
passages in his writings shew an insight into what chemistry
might ultimately accomplish, most of the chemical explanations of physiological phenomena so far put forward were
treated by him with contempt. He saw his way clear so long
as he was dealing with the size and shape of particles, and was

loth to leave these for unmeasurable and occult qualities. Malpighi seems to have been in his younger days much drawn towards chemical studies, but the more exact results of microscopical inquiry soon carried him too far away from them. Stensen more than any of the men whom we have mentioned in the preceding lectures recognized the part which chemistry might in the future play in the progress of physiology, but he did not of himself contribute to the advance of the infant science. Chemical physiology had an origin of its own and for a long time advanced on a line of its own, separate from or even antagonistic to other branches of physiology. To this we must now turn.

At the close of the fifteenth century, in the year 1493, according to some 1490, twenty years or more before the birth of Vesalius, there was born at the little town Maria Einsiedeln near the Lake of Zug, in the Canton of Schwyz, in Switzerland (whither to quite a late period pilgrimages were made), one who, under the name of Paracelsus, achieved a reputation more widely recognized in succeeding times than that of any of the names which I have hitherto mentioned, that perhaps of Harvey alone excepted.

His real name was Theophrastus Bombast von Hohenheim; to this others have added the words Philippus Aureolus; but he always called himself Theophrastus von Hohenheim. His father Wilhelm von Hohenheim was a physician at Einsiedeln, and his mother had a position in the hospital there; scandal alleges that he was the natural son of a person of high degree. The name Paracelsus is supposed by some to be a punning translation of Hohenheim; others maintain that he himself adopted it as indicating that he was a greater than Celsus. While he was quite young, in 1502, his father moved to Villach in Carinthia and there he seems to have spent some of his early days. He is said, at the age of sixteen, to have entered the University of Basel, but soon afterwards to have become the pupil of the Bishop Trithemius at Würzburg. Later on he appears to have spent some time in some mines in the Tyrol which were owned by the family Fugger. His personal history, however, especially in his earlier years, is wrapt in much uncertainty.

It would not be fitting to the purpose which I have in hand to dwell at length on the life and doings of this remarkable, this picturesque man, whose name has become a by-word for fantastic thought and even for charlatanry. But for the understanding of the genesis of chemical physiology it is necessary to say a few words about him.

To understand Paracelsus and his work we must, however, go back to a man of still a generation before. In the latter half of the fifteenth century there lived at Erfurt a Benedictine monk, of whose personal life little is known, one Basil Valentine, whose writings, the principal one of which was his *Currus triumphalis antimonii*, teach us chiefly what can be learnt about him.

He was one of the alchemists; but in addition to his inquiries into the properties of metals and his search for the philosopher's stone he busied himself with the nature of drugs, vegetable and mineral, and with their action as remedies for disease. He was no anatomist, no physiologist, but rather what nowadays we should call a pharmacologist. He did not care for the problems of the body, all he sought to understand was how the constituents of the soil and of plants might be treated so as to be available for healing the sick, and how they produced their effects. We apparently owe to him the introduction of many chemical substances, for instance of hydrochloric acid, which he prepared from oil of vitriol and salt, and of many vegetable drugs. And he apparently was the author of certain conceptions which as we shall see played an important part in the development of chemistry and of physiology. To him it seems we owe the idea of the three 'elements,' as they were and have been called, replacing the old idea of the ancients of the four elements, earth, air, fire and water. It must be remembered, however, that both in the ancient and in the new idea the word 'element' was not intended to mean that which it means to us now, a fundamental unit of matter, but a general quality or property of matter. The three elements of Valentine were (1) sulphur, or that which is combustible, which is changed or destroyed, or which at all events disappears during burning or combustion, (2) mercury, that which temporarily disappears, which is dissociated in burning from the body burnt, but which may be recovered, that is to say, that which is volatile, and (3) salt, that which is fixed, the residue or ash which remains after burning.

To understand the beginnings of chemical physiology it is important to remember the meanings attached to these three words. In Valentine's mind, and long, long after him sulphur did not mean the particular substance of a yellow colour, with distinct atomic weight and other qualities which we now call sulphur, but simply the constituent of any body, mineral, vegetable, or animal, which disappeared and was apparently wholly lost on burning. And so with mercury and salt.

To this conception of the properties of matter Valentine added one concerning the forces which govern and determine the phenomena of the universe, chemical changes included. He spoke of an *archaeus*, or of several *archaei*, as being instruments by which the Ruler of the Universe brought about events; these were to him the embodiments of energy.

Paracelsus was early introduced into alchemical studies while he was studying under the Bishop Trithemius; he probably learnt from him the doctrines of Valentine. These seem to have taken firm possession of his mind before he entered upon the ordinary medical studies of the time. It may be noted that those who were engaged in the search for the philosopher's stone and on the attendant chemical inquiries were, as a rule, not doctors, and carried on their work apart from the universities and medical schools. Many, very many of them were monks, or at least ecclesiastics, and pursued their investigations in solitude and retirement. A certain antagonism arose between this nascent science of chemistry and that older biological learning which formed the basis of medical education. The latter was the heritage of a long-established, powerful profession; the former was the product of amateurs, of the efforts of scattered independent workers, and as such was despised by professional men.

We know little as to the extent to which Paracelsus carried out his strictly medical, his anatomical and other studies; but it is clear that whether he learnt much or little, the knowledge which he thus gained was, even in view of medical practice, of little account in his mind compared with the new chemical science of which the doctors knew so little. He prized the knowledge which had come to him through the alchemical teaching of Trithemius, in the mines of Tyrol and in his subsequent wanderings as of more value than anything which he could learn from the expositors of Galen. Hence when after some years of travel, in which he is said to have wandered away in the East as far as Samarcand, ever seeking it would appear new chemical knowledge, he settled in 1527 as a physician at Basel, it was not to be wondered that he came into conflict with his orthodox brethren.

He may have been the turbulent, disorderly, noisy combative fellow that he is represented to be: often deep in his cups, and always, whether drunk or sober, ready to shout aloud that his opponent was an ignorant fool and idiot, and that he alone held the keys of truth. Even if he had not been this, if he had been quiet, modest, and shrinking, he had laid hold of something which the ordinary doctors of his time ignored and despised, the beginning of that chemical knowledge which in later years was to become one of the foundations of their science, and the mainstay of their art. And this was enough to put him in antagonism with them.

Driven away from Basel by their united opposition, he wandered forth from place to place carrying with him his scholars, his chemical apparatus, and his turbulent preaching of his new doctrines. Now rising on the flood of success, with what seemed the no less than marvellous cure of some sick great man whom the orthodox doctors had given up to death, now plunged into some ignoble quarrel and hard pressed with penury, never staying long in one spot, true to nothing but to the assertion of his own ideas, he ended at Salzburg in 1541, just as Vesalius was finishing his great work, his strange pilgrim life, by what is generally credited to have been a violent death in a drunken brawl.

The doctrines which he taught with such intemperate zeal were as I have said in the main the doctrines of Valentine, but enlarged, and developed by the new light which he had gained by his own researches and studies. He discovered many new chemical bodies, and introduced many new remedies. He had a great hand in the spread of that drug, which perhaps more than any one drug has influenced the fortunes of mankind, namely laudanum, the use of which is said to have been due to him. He was emphatically not an anatomist, not a physiologist, but a pharmacologist. He paid little heed to the doctrines of Galen, and cared little or nothing for anatomy. He was a chemist to the backbone; and his pathology was based not on changes of structure and their attendant symptoms but on the relation of diseases to drugs. He insisted that diseases ought to be known by the names of the drugs which cured them, *morbus helleborinus*, and the like; in this he was a forerunner of an errant school of therapeutics in modern times.

His physiology, if we may so call it, may perhaps as part of his philosophy be briefly described as follows:

Nature consists of visible matter and invisible forces. The visible matter is constituted of the three elements, sulphur, mercury, and salt; and attached to matter are forces, or perhaps we should say properties, by which changes of matter are brought about. But over and above these material forces or properties, matter is subject to and its changes are governed by spiritual forces, prominent among which are the *archaei*, "the chief *archaeus* being that exalted invisible spirit, that "occult virtue which is the artificer of nature in everyone."

All physiological processes, according to him, are chemical processes governed by the *archaeus*. In health, all the varied chemical processes are rightly governed by the *archaeus*. Death is the loss of the *archaeus*, the natural chemical changes being then left entirely to themselves. Disease is the failure of the *archaeus* to govern aright, and is often the result of the entrance into the body of germs bringing about chemical changes which the *archaeus* cannot master.

From this basis of philosophy there naturally followed his system of therapeutics, which consisted on the one hand in drugs which by their chemical properties assist the *archaeus* in its struggles with chemical changes, and on the other in occult invisible spiritual agencies, magnetic, astral and the like (for the stars working through the *archaei* affect the chemical processes of the body) which more directly join hands with the *archaeus*.

Paracelsus' doctrines as he put them forward had little or nothing in common with either the Galenic teaching of the day or the anatomical teaching of the succeeding age. They stood outside these, and seemed to such men as Vesalius and his followers the ravings of an ignorant charlatan. Nevertheless after a time, after the lapse of nearly a hundred years, they were taken up by a man, who so handled them that in a modified and developed shape they found lodgement in ordinary medical teaching and served as the starting-point of that chemical investigation of the problems of living beings which since that time and especially in these later years has been so fruitful of results. As Paracelsus, with the aid of some fifty years of increased knowledge, extended and developed Valentine's ideas so his doctrines were in turn extended and developed with the aid of a hundred years of increased knowledge (and those hundred years were as we have seen rich beyond measure in intellectual gains) by van Helmont, to whom we must now turn.

Jean Baptiste van Helmont was born at Brussels in 1577, some thirty odd years after Paracelsus' death, and more than ten years after that of Vesalius. His father died when he was three years old, and his mother, who was of one of the best Belgian families, took much care of his education, sending him at seventeen years of age to study philosophy at Louvain, which university was still of great repute. The teachers there however, eminent though they were, failed to satisfy the intellectual longings and the acute mind of the young van Helmont. To him their sayings seemed empty words; they made a great pretence to learning, but in what they taught he could see no real truth, could find no satisfaction for his mind. He refused to take the degree of Master of Arts, as being a sign of scholastic frippery, not of real knowledge. Anxious to satisfy his thirst for truth, he turned to systematic botany, beginning, at that period, to be seriously studied; but this in turn he found to be as dry and as unsatisfying as the herbaria which supplied its means of study. He then tried law, but this he soon found worse than even the others. He had almost reached the stage of Faust,

> Habe nun, ach! Philosophie
> Juristerei und—

But he had not yet tried medicine. This he was led to do, and in this he, for the first time, found what his soul desired. I mention these earlier ventures of his because they are indications of an acute active mind earnestly seeking after real truth; and love of truth, in spite of the somewhat fantastic form which his ideas, after the fashion of Paracelsus, took in his later writings, was after all the key-note of his character.

He threw himself so heartily into his medical studies that in 1599, at the early age of twenty-two, he took his Doctorship of Medicine, and is said to have been appointed immediately afterwards to deliver a course of lectures on surgery.

Wisely however he decided to travel, and the next four or five years he spent in visiting different countries, Switzerland, Italy (where he is said to have met Fabricius), France, and England.

Returning home in 1605, he arrived in time to study the great epidemic of plague then raging in Antwerp, and afterwards settled for a while at Brussels; later in 1609, having married a rich heiress, he took up his abode in the neighbouring town of Vilvorde. Here he remained for the remainder of his life, practising to a certain extent as a physician, chiefly however it would appear as a work of charity, for his means were ample, but mainly occupied with carrying out chemical observations and experiments. And here in 1644 he died.

He published several books, the first in 1617; but his ideas and doctrines are chiefly embodied in his work *Ortus Medicinae*, which however did not see the light until 1648, four years after his death, being edited by his son.

He was as we shall see a devout Catholic, an obedient son of the Church; nevertheless a work which he published in 1621, *De Magnetica Vulnerum Curatione*, in which insisting as Paracelsus had done on the potency of magnetic virtues he seemed to explain away, on physical grounds, some of the miracles, he came into conflict with the spiritual powers; and for some time during the latter part of his life was condemned to imprisonment, though his own house was allowed to serve as his gaol.

Van Helmont, as I have already hinted, was from a certain point of view a Paracelsus, a modest, softened Paracelsus come to life again, but come again to a quite different world.

The medical studies, in which van Helmont first found something solid to rest upon, were not the vague Galenic teachings which were all that had been offered to Paracelsus, but teachings based on the exact anatomical knowledge provided by Vesalius and his school, and on all which that knowledge carried with it. So soon as he had graduated, perhaps even while he was still a student, there came to him as to all others in Northern Europe some of that new, exact physical learning which was starting up in Pisa and in Padua. While he was engaged in his own labours, long before he had completed them, twenty years before his death, Harvey's great work was open before him. He must have heard of it; but it may be doubted whether he ever read it. Certainly he was not convinced by Harvey's arguments, for in his writings, though he combats several of the Galenic doctrines concerning the heart, he still accepts the Galenic view of the passage of the blood from the right side of the heart to the left through the pores of the septum. Still eight years earlier, in 1620, there had appeared the *Novum Organon* of Francis Bacon, which, though it probably had no influence on van Helmont and most likely had never been seen by him, was a characteristic product of the time and at least shewed the tenor of the thoughts among which he lived. It is more than probable that he might have met Descartes, or have read his *Discours de la Méthode* published in 1637. And he must have been aware of the discovery of the lacteals by Aselli in 1622.

The things of science were very different in the first quarter of the seventeenth from what they were in the first quarter of the sixteenth century, in which Paracelsus lived. And much of the new learning had sunk deep into van Helmont's mind. Yet for all that it was Paracelsus above all others who seems to have influenced his thoughts. As you read his *Ortus Medicinae* you are struck by the fact that while he rarely if ever mentions the great names of which I have spoken, Vesalius and the rest, the name of Paracelsus and the mention of Paracelsus' views occur again and again; moreover the main doctrines which he develops are Paracelsus' doctrines in a new dress.

Yet at the same time it must be confessed that as we read van Helmont we seem to see two men, two intellects of very different kinds.

On the one hand we see a patient, careful, exact observer, a child of the new philosophy, one who has entered fully into the spirit of the new physics, who watches, measures and weighs, who takes advantage of the aid of instruments of exact research, who reaches a conclusion by means of accurate quantitative estimations. On the other hand we see a mystic, speculative dreamer, a philosopher in the old sense of the word, one weaving a fantastic scheme of the powers and forces ruling the universe, calling in the aid of invisible supernatural agencies to explain the occurrence of natural phenomena. And throughout the whole of his writings is seen the continued endeavour to weave his exact chemical physical knowledge and his spiritualistic views into a consistent whole. Again and again he refers to instances of the former as proofs or illustrations of the latter.

These two sides of van Helmont's character are not unfitly indicated by the two words *Gas* and *Blas*, 'two new terms,' he himself says, "introduced by me because a knowledge of them "(*i.e.* of the things which they indicate) was hidden from the "ancients."

By '*Blas*' he meant, so far as can be ascertained, the same thing as the *archaeus* of Paracelsus. It is true he uses the word *archaeus* as if he meant by it something different from *Blas*, but he often seems to use the one or the other indifferently. In any case he believed as did Paracelsus in an invisible spiritual or at least immaterial agency or energy which directed and governed material processes and changes. He speaks of a *Blas meteoron* which governs the heavens, and of a *Blas humanum* which presides over and determines all the functions of the human body. The events of the human body according to him as according to Paracelsus are governed by an *archaeus*, or rather by a hierarchy of minor *archaei*, all subject to and ministrants of the chief *archaeus*. There is a *Blas motivum* presiding over movements, and a *Blas altera-*

tivum presiding over what we now call metabolic changes; and the *Blas motivum* is dual, for there is a *Blas* which presides over voluntary and a *Blas* which presides over natural movements. And there are other special kinds of *Blas*.

But if by *Blas* van Helmont shews himself something not very different from a Paracelsus redivivus, by *Gas* he clearly disentangles himself from all the mystic Paracelsean lore, and earns for himself the title of the first of modern chemists, and at the same time the first of chemical physiologists.

By *Gas* he clearly meant, and by the introduction of the new term indicates his appreciation of the discovery of, what we now call carbonic acid gas, or carbon dioxide; and, as we shall see, the development of a great deal of chemistry, and especially of the chemistry of living beings, has turned on the nature and properties of gases.

It was in relation to this gas that he parts company with Paracelsus. He argues that Paracelsus was wholly wrong in maintaining that sulphur, mercury, and salt were the three elements. There are he contends two elements only, air, that is to say the natural atmosphere, and water. He spends much time in proving that air and water can never be changed, the one into the other, that they are distinct and never convertible, that the vapour of water is something wholly different from real air.

On the other hand, by what he called water he meant everything which is not air; he insists that all things, plants and animals, can be reduced to water, that they are in fact water endued with certain properties.

"That all vegetables and flesh consist of water alone I can "prove by experiment. Everything indeed if not directly, at "least with the help of an adjunct, can be made to assume "again the nature of water. All stones, rocks and mud, either "of themselves, or with assistance, change into alkaline salt "(sal alkali); and all sal alkali, fat being added, is reduced to "a watery liquor which at length becomes plain and simple "water."

Here is an example of the quantitative method by which he carried out his investigations:

"That all vegetables are produced immediately and
"materially out of the single element of water I learnt by
"experiment. I took an earthen vessel in which I placed
"200 lbs. of earth dried in an oven. I then watered it with
"rain water and planted in it a young willow weighing 16 lbs.
"After the expiration of five years this willow weighed 169 lbs.
"and some ounces.

"The earthen vessel, which was always, when necessary,
"moistened with rain or with distilled water, was large, and
"was sunk in the ground; and lest any dust carried by the
"air should be mingled with the earth, an iron lid coated
"with tin closed the mouth of the vessel. I did not measure
"the weight of the leaves which were shed in the four suc-
"cessive autumns. At the end, I dried the earth in the vessel,
"and found its weight to be 200 lbs. less some two ounces.

"The 164 lbs. or so of wood, bark, and roots (by which the
"older tree differed in weight from the young one) were
"therefore derived from water alone."

Is not this a good experiment, one such as an experimental
agricultural station of to-day need not be ashamed of? It is
only the conclusion that is wrong. Would not van Helmont be
now delighted to hear that it was not water but gas, carbon
dioxide, which in the main accounted for the increase in
weight?

He goes on to expound how out of many things can be
obtained, in various ways, a something which is like air, but
is not air, not the air of the atmosphere. This appears when
wood is burnt, when the must of grapes or of malt ferments
in the making of wine or beer, and on other occasions; and
this he calls 'gas.'

He gives it that name, because the sound is not so far from
that of 'chaos,' the unformed womb of all things.

Here is an experiment giving a quantitative proof of the
existence of gas in wood or charcoal:

"Charcoal moreover, even if heated in a closed vessel for
"nine days in a burning furnace, though it is exposed to
"combustion—for the fire has access to the charcoal in the
"closed vessel just as it does when charcoal is burnt in the
"open—nevertheless is not at all consumed. It cannot be

"consumed because its effluvium is prevented. Charcoal there-
"fore, and we may say generally all things which do not
"directly change into water, and are not fixed, necessarily
"give forth the spirit of wood (spiritum sylvestre). Consider
"that of 62 lbs. of charcoal of oak, 1 lb. only remains as ash
"when it is burnt. The remaining 61 lbs. therefore consist of
"that spirit of wood which, even though the charcoal be
"exposed to fire, cannot escape from a closed vessel. This
"spirit, hitherto unknown, I call by the name of 'gas.' * * *
"Many bodies indeed contain this spirit, and some are
"wholly changed into it. Not indeed that it is present in these
"in its actual state of gas, but as a condensed spirit, solidified
"to suit the fashion of the body in which it resides; and it
"may be set free by the action of a ferment as in wine or
"bread."

This idea of a ferment setting free gas by its action was one
of which, as we shall see, he made great use. He says:

"A grape uninjured may be dried and kept without change
"for an indefinite time; but if once its skin be broken, it
"presently receives the ferment of ebullition, and hence the
"beginning of change.

"The juice of grapes, apples, berries, honey, and even
"bruised flowers and twigs, a ferment having been laid hold
"of, begin to bubble and effervesce, whence gas.

"When I was a student, misled by the authority of ignorant
"writers, I thought that the gas of grapes was the spirit of
"wine in the must; but negative experiments shewed me that
"the gas of grapes and must was preparatory to the wine but
"not the spirit of wine (alcohol) itself.

"The history of gas is well shewn by gunpowder, which
"consists of saltpetre, sulphur and charcoal. When these are
"mixed together and ignited there is no vessel in nature which
"(if these were shut up in it) would not, on account of the gas
"produced, burst."

His gas he affirms is not air. "Some impostors think that
"gas is wind or air occluded in things, having been introduced
"into the mixture of elements at the origin of things." But
this is not so. Gas is really a form of water. "The gas of
"salts is water. That the gas of fruits is nothing but water

"follows from what I have already shewn, namely, that these
"arise from water. A dried grape, submitted to distillation,
"is thereby reduced by art to elemental water, whereas a
"grape fresh but injured gives rise to must and gas. Since
"therefore the whole grape in the absence of ferment is turned
"into water, but gives rise to gas whenever a ferment is
"applied, it follows of necessity that the gas is itself water."

Deeply impressed with this idea of the action of ferments,
van Helmont makes it the basis of his system of physiology.
Nearly all the writers before him had caught hold of the
phenomena of the fermenting wine-vat, as being, though
mysterious in themselves, illustrative of the still more
mysterious phenomena of the living body; and the old idea
of the physiological spirits of the body, natural, vital and
animal, was connected in its origin with this same formation
of alcohol, of spirits of wine by fermentation. The anatomical
school of Vesalius and those after him, busy with other things,
did not attempt to develop the conception; they, as we have
seen, passed on one side of the chemical events of the living
body. Van Helmont was the first to attempt a connected
exposition of these matters. He was doubtless well acquainted
with the physiological and anatomical teaching of the time.
But in his writings he dwells very little on these; he is chiefly
concerned with the chemical events which others had neglected.

His exposition of physiology is based on a theory of fermentations. The ordinary vinous fermentation gives him his
initial idea; following this up, he regards all the changes in
the body (not digestion only but also all others including
nutrition, impregnation and even movement) as due to the
action of ferments. And he reconciles this view with his view
of the influence of the *Blas* or *Archaeus*, by the hypothesis
that these spiritual agents work not by acting directly on
matter, but by making use of the ferments, which are thus
their servants or instruments. The following is a brief sketch
of his exposition of physiological events:

He assumes the current teaching of the day to be (1) that
the food absorbed from the stomach and intestine is in the
liver endued with natural spirits, (2) that in the heart the

natural spirits are converted into vital spirits, and (3) that in
the brain the vital spirits are converted into animal spirits.
And indeed this was still to a large extent the teaching of the
day. It was, as we have seen, the exposition given by Descartes
even after van Helmont's death; the influence of the Harveian
doctrines had not as yet made themselves fully felt.

All this current teaching, says van Helmont, is wrong.
There are not three conversions, three upward developments
only, but in reality six. And each of these upward steps is of
the nature of a fermentation; he speaks of them as six
digestions or concoctions, by which the dead food becomes
the living, active flesh.

The *first* stage is the digestion in the stomach. It may be
noted that he wholly ignores saliva and the changes in the
mouth; Steno and Wharton had not yet written. It is obvious,
he says, that in the stomach food and drink are converted into
chyle; and this conversion takes place by means of a ferment.
But this ferment does not reside permanently in the stomach,
is not always there, for digestion is not continually going on
in the stomach; the process is an intermittent one. The
ferment really comes from the spleen; it is from the spleen
that the stomach draws all its energy. And in another part
of his book he dwells on what he calls the duumvirate, the
dual reign of the stomach and the spleen. He was still under
the dominion of the old traditions of the spleen; he had not
got so far even as the clear-sighted Vesalius; and Malpighi
had not yet written. This ferment in the stomach is an acid
ferment (questions of acids, alkalis and salts were beginning
to move the chemists of the time); but the acidity is not the
ferment itself, is only the organ or instrument of the ferment.
"If the ferment were only an acid, vinegar alone would be
"able to transmute a mass of bread and be sufficient for the
"transformation of all our food." He adds that "condiments
"help digestion, not because they add to the ferment, for
"a ferment can add nothing to itself, it is a specific gift of
"vital nature; they simply prepare the food for the easier
"access of the ferment."

In this exposition of peptic digestion we recognize the
careful, exact observer; for the above comes very near to the

doctrines of to-day, and even the idea about the spleen has its modern analogue.

He then goes on to state that the acid chyle, passing into the duodenum, immediately acquires a saline nature, changes from an acid into a salt, "just as vinegar by the addition of "nimium (lead oxide) is changed into an aluminous sweetness." But this analogy is, he hastens to say, a lame one. The change in the duodenum is brought about 'through a more excellent vigour of transmutation.' The ferment actions of which he is speaking are much more complicated than ordinary chemical actions. It is, I may say in passing, worth while to note this expression; it shews that van Helmont was nearer the truth than some of those who immediately followed him.

This change in the duodenum constitutes van Helmont's *second digestion*, and the ferment by which it is effected is furnished by the bile; he argues at great length that the bile is not a mere excrement, but is or contains a ferment. And he remarks in passing that the work of the acid ferment of the stomach ceases when the chyle reaches the duodenum. "For "every ferment dislikes to have as its allies things foreign to "itself; it will not listen to the commands of strange masters, "it refuses to play the thief and put its sickle into another's "harvest." We repeat this saying of van Helmont's, when to-day we teach that the pepsin of the stomach is destroyed in the duodenum by the bile and pancreatic juice. Of pancreatic juice van Helmont knew nothing, for Wirsung had as yet not written.

The *third digestion* to which this duodenal digestion, by which as we sometimes now say acid chyme is converted into alkaline chyle, is the prelude, is that of sanguification, which beginning in the mesenteric veins is continued in the liver, and completed in the vena cava, a sanguification by which the chyle is converted into blood, into crude blood, into cruor and into serum, not yet into vivified blood; the cruor will later on become this vivified blood, the serum being used for the formation of urine and of sweat.

The ferment for this third digestion is furnished by the liver, which thus supplies two ferments. One is carried to the duodenum by the bile from the gall-bladder; and it almost seems as if van Helmont accepted the view that was held by some that the bile was secreted by the gall-bladder and not by the liver itself. The other descends from the liver along the mesenteric veins. And he notes that the sanguification of chyle, its conversion into blood being a more exquisite digestion than the acid fermentation of food into chyle, takes place, not like that in one wide open cavity but in a number of narrow, and yet not too narrow, passages.

It is worthy of notice that van Helmont, though well acquainted as he obviously was with the medical literature of the day, little as he might esteem some of it, and therefore probably aware of Aselli's discovery, makes no mention of lacteals. He regards all the chyle as being absorbed by the veins; and argues that since the chyle is not ready for absorption until it has been prepared by the second duodenal digestion there is no real absorption of food from the stomach.

He has his views about the mechanism of absorption. He relates an experiment to shew that salts dissolved in water will pass through a membrane such as a pig's bladder; and he contends that absorption of chyle takes place partly in the same way that salts pass through membranes, by diffusion as we should now say, and partly by minute orifices in the walls of the intestine, orifices which while open during life are closed at death so that no absorption is possible from a dead intestine.

The refuse of the food, left after the absorption of the nutritious chyle, passing along the intestine, meets in the caecum with a stercoraceous ferment by which it is converted into faeces.

Such in brief outline is van Helmont's story of what even now-a-days we sometimes call primary and secondary digestion.

The *fourth digestion* takes place in the heart and arteries. By this elaboration the darker and thicker blood of the vena cava becomes lighter in colour and distinctly volatile. By this he obviously means the change from venous to arterial blood. But he does not very clearly distinguish between this fourth digestion and his succeeding *fifth digestion*, "which changes "the blood of the arteries into the vital spirit of the *archaeus*."

He distinguishes between the crude blood (cruor) supplied by the liver and the vitalized blood (sanguis) distributed by the heart through the arteries.

"I never could satisfy myself," says he, "that there was "any spirit in the crude blood (cruor) coming from the liver, "though this had already acquired its own grade of perfection "after it had left the mesentery. The crude blood from the "liver has always seemed to me mere material for use; it "ought not to be considered as perfect vital blood."

His view seems to be that by the time it reaches the arteries the crude material blood has become vitalized blood, through the presence of the *spiritus vitalis*. This spiritus is of the nature of or acts after the fashion of a ferment, it multiplies itself as a ferment does. It is always present on the left side of the heart, in the arterial blood of the left ventricle, and some of it is drawn through the septum, from the left side to the right, by minute pores which are too minute to allow blood to pass.

"Some of this spiritus," says he, "this ferment, thus drawn "through the septum begins to multiply even on the right side "of the heart. The right side of the heart labours incessantly "for no other end than that it should draw a little spiritus "from the left side across the septum of the heart in order "that the crude blood in the vena cava close to the heart "should by the participation of that spiritus at once begin "to be vivified."

Apparently the fourth digestion is only the beginning or a part of the fifth digestion, which as a whole consists in the vivification of the blood, the conversion of crude into vitalized blood by the addition and influence of the spiritus vitalis, always present in the left ventricle, always subject to multiplication and increase.

Two points may be noticed here. One is that van Helmont came very near to and yet wholly missed the use of air in breathing. The other is his singular clinging to the passage through the septum.

We have seen how, in spite of the direct evidence of their senses, men clung for centuries to the view that the blood passed through the solid septum of the heart, from the right to the left ventricle. In spite of Servetus' stout assertion that such a passage was impossible, in spite of Vesalius' biting sarcasms, in spite of Columbus and Caesalpinus the view still held its ground; it gave way before Harvey, not because Harvey like those before him denied it but because he shewed a better way. Van Helmont, Harvey's contemporary, born the year before him and dying twenty-three years before him, had not, as we have seen, profited by what Harvey had done; he still believed that the blood passed through the septum from the right to the left ventricle. He added to the old view a new one, that the fermentative spirit which vitalized the blood passed also through the septum, but in the contrary direction, namely from left to right. And he argued that the pits in the septum, being conical in shape with their narrow apices abutting on the left ventricle and their broad bases on the right ventricle, were so constructed in order that they might prevent the return of the blood itself from the left side to the right though they allowed the passage of the more subtle spirit. The story forms an odd page in the history of human thought, a page odd but full of warning. When we examine our own views to-day about this matter and that, are we sure that we are not asserting that things are passing through a septum though our senses shew us that there are in it no channels through which such a passage can take place?

And now comes a remarkable generalisation, by which van Helmont leaps ahead and anticipates conclusions which were not reached until many a long year after him.

"The sixth and last digestion takes place in the kitchens of "the several members, for there are as many stomachs as "there are nutritive members. In this sixth digestion a "spiritus, a ferment innate in each place, cooks its food for "itself." In the language of to-day, all the tissues live upon the common blood, and the power of assimilation lies in the tissue itself; it is the tissue and not the blood which primarily determines assimilation, the qualities of the blood have only an indirect influence. "A vein," says van Helmont, meaning probably an artery, "may be considered as a vessel con-"taining aliment prepared for the kitchens of the tissues, but

"it is not their kitchen. Each tissue maintains its own in-
"dividual kitchen within itself."

He gives as an instance the nutrition of muscle. Accepting
the as yet common view (Stensen and Borelli had not yet
written) that muscle consists of an inactive, passive, non-
contractile part, the 'caro,' or flesh, and the active contractile
part, the fibres, van Helmont suggests that the crude parts of
blood can directly, without elaborate nutritive action, supply
the 'caro,' the flesh, which therefore can at any time increase
and grow in a vegetative manner, but that the fibres are
nourished by the vivified blood, through the activity of the
tissue ferments, and the growth of this, the active part of
the muscle, is therefore subject to the laws of life.

A corollary to this view of the sixth digestion, of the action
of the individual ferments of the several tissues, is of no little
importance; it led van Helmont to a position far in advance
of his peers.

"I make," says he, "no distinction between vital and
"animal spirits. The same blood with the same vital spirits,
"vitalized blood (arterial blood as we should say), is carried
"to all the tissues. The boat has only one rudder, each tissue
"lives upon that blood, exercising its own functions, the brain
"and other nervous tissues behaving in this respect like the
"rest of the tissues. As the spiritus, the so-called animal
"spirit, does not differ specifically in itself in the several
"organs of senses and instruments of movement, though the
"senses and the movements differ among themselves, so it
"is unnecessary to suppose an animal spirit apart from the
"vital spirit of the vitalized blood."

So far I have dwelt upon van Helmont's work on what we
may call its rational side. What I have briefly described
constitutes a general exposition of the main facts of chemical
physiology, as van Helmont conceived them, and, as we have
seen, many of his conclusions were based on careful observations and indeed on experiment. That exposition exerted a
great influence on investigators coming after him. In the
first place it shewed that many of the problems of the living
body were chemical problems to be solved by chemical knowledge, not problems of a mechanical nature only, not problems

to be solved by the experimental verification of a suggestion offered by anatomical arrangements. In the second place it drew the attention of inquirers to the fact, which experience has shewn to be an undoubted fact, that a large number of the processes taking place in the living body are more or less akin to the process by which yeast produces alcohol, as in wine-making or brewing, and therefore may be spoken of as fermentations. This idea of the fermentative nature of the changes taking place in the living body was as we have said an old one, it had been preached by Paracelsus; but its definite introduction into physiological thought is due to van Helmont. The authors coming afterwards who dwelt on the subject all acknowledge their indebtedness to him. In the third place his discovery of carbonic acid gas, and of other gases, for he recognized that all gas was not alike, that some gas for instance was inflammable, was a chemical discovery of prime importance, though the value of the discovery did not become apparent until after the lapse of many years.

But to judge by his writings van Helmont was at heart more pleased with his Blas than with his Gas. In the exposition of which I have given an account there are repeated interpositions, which I have omitted, numerous references to the action of this or that blas or archaeus. And any attempt to picture van Helmont's mind would be incomplete without at least some few words about his views as to the relations of the archaeus, and so of the phenomena of the body, to what he calls the sensitive and motive soul, the *anima sensitiva motivaque*.

"This sensitive soul belongs to man alone; for speaking "truly and thinking correctly, we must say that there is no "soul residing in plants and in brute beasts. These possess "only a certain vital power, which we may perhaps regard as "the forerunner of a soul. The sensitive soul as it exists in "man takes to itself the reins of that forerunning governing "vital power, which thus melting into the archaeus submits "itself to the sensitive soul."

The sensitive soul is the prime agent of all the acts of the body, the archaeus being its servant, the minor archaei also its servants, and the ferments the instruments in turn of the archaei; it is this which is, among its other services, the prime

cause of the vital spirit which in the heart vitalizes the blood.
Though it carries out the sensations and movements of the
body by means of the brain and nerves, its actual throne is in
the pylorus; it resides in the orifice of the stomach. He gives
various reasons for this conclusion; among others the facts
that a great emotion is always felt at the pit of the stomach,
and that a man may have his head blown off by a cannon-ball
and yet his heart will go on beating for some time, whereas
a severe blow at the pit of the stomach will stop his heart and
take away his consciousness at the same time.

But the throne or temple of this sensitive soul is of a
peculiar nature. It is in the archaeus of the stomach that the
soul dwells; "there it sits and there it abides all life long."
"Not that the sensitive soul dwells in the stomach as in a sack,
"in a skin, in a membrane, in a bag, in a prison or in a shell.
"Nor is it confined to that seat after the fashion of things shut
"up in a purse. In a wholly peculiar manner is it present, in
"a point centrally, in an atom as it were, in the middle of the
"thickness of a mere membrane. Though it is placed in a
"locality, it is nevertheless not there in a local manner. For
"it is a light, and there is in the universe nothing so much
"like it as is the light of a candle; it is present in the stomach
"in some such way as light is present in a burning wick. But
"when I call it a light, I do not mean a burning, heating light,
"the cause of the heat of the body, for the heat of the body
"is merely the product of life, of vital actions, and is not life
"itself."

This sensitive soul is mortal, and in man, in his present
state, coexists with the immortal mind, *mens immortalis*, the
two being connected in a peculiar way. "The sensitive soul is
"as it were the husk or shell of the mind, and the latter works
"through it, so that at the bidding of the mind the soul makes
"use of the archaeus whether it itself will or no."

"Before the Fall of Adam man possessed only the im-
"mortal mind which acted directly on the archaeus, and while
"this was the case, while the immortal mind discharged all
"the functions of life, and the sensitive soul as yet was not,
"man was immortal, and the shadows of the brute beast did
"not blur his intellect.

"At the Fall God introduced into man the sensitive soul, "and with it death, the immortal mind retiring within the "sensitive soul and becoming as it were its kernel."

In thus speaking of these speculative flights of van Helmont by which he brought his chemical views as to the nature of man into harmony with the teaching of the Church, of which, in spite of the heresy attributed to him, he was a devoted son, I may seem to be travelling away from the proper province of physiology. And yet this theory of the sensitive soul did definitely enter into subsequent physiological thought. Both parts of van Helmont's teaching left their mark on succeeding inquiries and thought. The influence of his doctrine of fermentations may, as I have just said, be traced down even to the present time; but that doctrine was early stripped of its archaeal and other wrappings and soon took on the form of a sober chemical knowledge.

The doctrine of the sensitive soul was also taken up by some of his successors; it appeared and reappeared at intervals, now in more or less its original, now in a modified, form. And as we pass in review the succession of opinions as to the ultimate causes of the phenomena of living beings we may trace a genetic bond between van Helmont's picturesque and vivid idea of a sensitive soul, and the paler, fainter views of a vital principle held by some at the present day.

LECTURE VI

SYLVIUS AND HIS PUPILS. THE PHYSIOLOGY OF DIGESTION IN THE SEVENTEENTH CENTURY

I PROPOSE to devote the present Lecture to an account of some men of the seventeenth century who may be regarded as the successors of van Helmont in chemical physiology, at least in that part of it which concerns digestion. But, before doing so, I should like to turn aside for a while to say something about a man, who, in the very early years of that century, though he did not deal much with either the new chemical or the new physical ideas, yet by applying the chief instrument of physical inquiry, namely exact measurement, to the determination of chemical data opened up a line of inquiry which, unknown before him and not greatly used in the times after him, has in these later years been made to produce most valuable results.

Of the life of Sanctorius Sanctorius we know very little. He was born at Capo d' Istria in 1561, he studied and graduated at Padua, and after travelling a good deal practised for some time in Venice. He was later on called to be professor of theoretical medicine in the University of Padua, where he gave a discourse in 1612, and where he achieved much fame, drawing many students to his lectures. After a while however he withdrew again to private practice in Venice, in which city he died in 1636.

In 1614 he published at Venice a small book entitled *Medical Statics*, which subsequently passed through many editions and was translated into several languages. It is composed of several hundred short aphorisms, dealing with air and water, with food and drink, with sleeping and waking and other like topics. Each aphorism is a deduction from facts determined by most careful measurements of the weight of his body at different times, of his food and of his excretions. But he gives no account whatever of his experiments; in striking contrast to many a modern memoir which seems in great measure hardly more than a transcript of laboratory notes, or at least consists in large part of detailed 'protocols' of experiments, Sanctorius' work gives only the bare conclusions. He merely describes in a very general way the method by which he arrived at his results. He had constructed a chair suspended to a steelyard, so that he could, using this as a balance, accurately determine his body-weight, at various times and under various conditions; and his book contains a quaint picture illustrating how he weighed himself before and after a meal. By this means he was able accurately to measure the loss of weight to his body by insensible perspiration. As he says in his Preface, "It is a new and unheard-of thing in "Medicine that anyone should be able to arrive at an exact "measurement of insensible perspiration. Nor has anyone "either Philosopher or Physician dared to attack this part of "medical inquiry. I am indeed the first to make the trial, "and unless I am mistaken I have by reasoning and by the "experience of thirty years brought this branch of science to "perfection, which I judged more advisable than to describe "all the details of my inquiry."

In his aphorisms he occasionally gives us glimpses of his experimental results, as when he says, "If the food and drink "in one day amount to eight pounds, the insensible transpira- "tion will generally amount to about five pounds"; but as I have said, the book consists in the main of deductions con- cerning changes taking place in the body as the result of this or that condition, the nature of the changes being inferred from data furnished by the amount of the insensible perspira- tion in relation to the weight of the food and drink, of the sensible evacuations and of the body. Sanctorius thus stands out as the forerunner in the early years of the seventeenth century of that statical method of physiological inquiry which during the latter half of the nineteenth century has produced such useful results. But he cared more for practical guidance than for theoretical conclusions. He regarded his balance as a means of helping a man 'to live according to rule.' He proposed that each meal should be taken sitting in his chair with the steelyard so adjusted that by the descent of the chair the diner should be warned that the predetermined weight of food had been swallowed. He was obviously a singularly original man; we learn for instance that he in- vented a thermometer for measuring the heat of the animal body, and an instrument for measuring the movements of the arteries.

We must however now return to the successors of van Helmont.

In 1614, the year before van Helmont wrote his first book and fourteen years before Malpighi's birth, there was born at Hanover of a good family one François De la Boe or Dubois, better known perhaps by his Latin name as Franciscus Sylvius. He is the second prominent man of that name in the history of physiology, the first being Jacobus Sylvius of Paris, in the sixteenth century, the teacher of Vesalius. Though a man of a wholly different type of intellect from van Helmont, Sylvius appears in the history of physiological thought as his legitimate descendant.

After studying at Sédan, at Basel, where in 1637 he took his degree, and elsewhere, and after a stay of some years at Amsterdam he became in 1658 Professor of Medicine at Leyden, and there for many years exerted a most powerful influence until his death in 1672.

In order to understand the importance and bearing of his physiological and medical teaching, the nature of which may be learnt from his many medical and physiological writings, it must be borne in mind that he was not only a physician and a physiologist, but also distinctly and clearly what we should now call a chemist. He published many purely chemical works. He persuaded the Curators of the University of Leyden to build for him a 'Laboratorium, as they call it'; this seems to have been the first University Chemical Laboratory.

Like Glauber, an older man, born in 1604 and dying in 1668, whose name is perpetuated in his sal mirabile, Glauber's salt, sodium sulphate, and who though he made no marked contribution to physiology, largely increased the chemical knowledge of his time, Sylvius devoted much energy to the study of salts. He probably owed much to Glauber, who appears to have been one of the first to lay hold of the idea of chemical affinity. But in any case Sylvius learnt to recognize the nature of many salts as the result of a union of acids with bases. He was the first to prove the presence of volatile alkalis in plants. And it is perhaps mainly by the increased knowledge of the various salts, and their composition, that his chemical science is in advance of that of van Helmont, who died just about or rather just before the time when Sylvius began to write.

If he was like van Helmont in being a chemist and in looking at the phenomena of life from a chemical point of view, and if he followed van Helmont in explaining many of the events of the living body as due to fermentative processes, and in this respect may be regarded as van Helmont's successor, he differed from him widely in almost every other respect. Van Helmont paid little heed to that part of physiology which is derived by deductions from anatomy, by experiments on animals or by the application of mechanical principles; Sylvius was well versed in all these things and wrote well on the circulation of the blood and on the mechanics of respiration. Harvey's teaching had apparently no influence on van Helmont; it entered largely into Sylvius's thoughts, and indeed it was chiefly through his advocacy that the Harveian doctrines became established in Holland. Van Helmont's mind was a double one, bent on the one hand on exact careful experiment, turned wistfully on the other hand to mystic speculations about invisible agencies and spirits. Sylvius shared the former mental attitude; the latter was wholly foreign to his character. Van Helmont was essentially an inquirer, most of his time was spent in his own home, pursuing his own researches; he cared more for following out his own ideas than for influencing the opinions of others. Sylvius was essentially an expositor; his own special contributions to the advancement of physiological, as distinguished from chemical, knowledge were unimportant. He was the discoverer of no new striking piece of physiological truth, unless perhaps it be the distinction between conglomerate and conglobate glands, to which we have already referred, and we owe to him it is true, and not to his older namesake, the aqueduct of Sylvius; but the new things which he made known were in the main chemical. Yet he occupies a not inconspicuous place in the history of physiology on account of his power and enthusiasm as a teacher. He became the founder of a school.

We may infer something about the influence of Sylvius as a teacher and about the scope of his teaching from what his brilliant pupil Stensen says of him. Towards the end of his larger treatise on muscle, Stensen, treating of what yet remained to be learnt about muscle, writes as follows:—

"No one as yet, so far as I know, has so joined Chemistry "to Anatomy as to have clearly and distinctly explained, not "by deductions from the doctrines of the schools but by "following up the indications of Nature, in what respects "muscle tendon and bone agree and in what they differ.

"My most eminent teacher Sylvius has laboured in this "way with happy results, in respect to the humours of our "body; and, if I remember rightly, I have often listened to "him while he, led by the same spirit of inquiry, discoursed "also concerning the nature of tendons and of bones. But that "eminent man although he has done much in this branch of "knowledge is, lest he might seem to sacrifice the public weal "to his own glory, in the habit of daily assuring his pupils "that he has not been able to accomplish everything. Hence "he expounds, in the shape of views and speculations, matters "concerning which he has not yet arrived at a clear and de-"finite result, and thus he stimulates others to inquiry, sup-"plying them at the same time with problems to begin with."

We learn from this that Sylvius had his mind open towards all the chemical problems presented by the human body, but that he busied himself chiefly with, and was most successful in, the study of the fluids of the body, the blood, the lymph and the several juices or secretions.

Sylvius as I have said followed van Helmont in considering a large number of the changes taking place in the living body as being of the nature of fermentative processes; but his idea of fermentation was a different one from that of van Helmont. The latter taking vinous fermentation as the type saw in the ferment which produced the change a subtle agency, having characters of its own, one whose effects were wholly different in kind from ordinary chemical events, from the result for instance of adding a base, such as lead oxide, to an acid, such as vinegar. The action of the ferment was in van Helmont's eyes of a more exquisite nature than a simple chemical change; the bubbles of gas which appeared in the fermenting vat were incidental things, not features essential to the action of the ferment. Sylvius saw nothing of all these subtle distinctions. To him the rising of the bubbles of gas, without the intervention of an extrinsic blast of air, seemed to be one of the essential facts of fermentation; and since he saw the same spontaneous escape of gas when an acid was poured over an earth or a salt, when oil of vitriol for instance was poured over chalk, he concluded that the two processes were identical in kind. Hence, though he continued often to use the word 'fermentation,' he more often used the word 'effervescence,' and at times seems to use the one or the other quite indifferently.

Vieussens, who, in addition to the researches in anatomy which have handed down to us the terms 'valve of Vieussens' and 'annulus of Vieussens,' busied himself with chemical matters, writing in 1688, *De natura etc. Fermentationis*, thus formally defines the various kinds of fermentation:

"Fermentation is the adventitious and expansive move-"ment of heterogeneous parts and of insensible fermenting "bodies excited without sensible cause, which, when it is "vehement or of long duration, brings about an essential "change or a conspicuous alteration in the fermenting bodies "themselves.

. "*Latent* fermentation, than which nothing is more common "alike in the works of nature and of man, is an adventitious "and expansive movement of heterogeneous parts and insen-"sible bodies excited without sensible cause, which, when it "is vehement or of long duration, brings about an essential "change or a conspicuous alteration in the fermenting bodies "themselves and is excited so gradually and in so hidden a "manner that while it is taking place it can not be detected "by the senses, and hence is only recognized by the effects "which in a given time it produces.

"Of this kind is the movement of the particles of a mass of "dough which is beginning to ferment, but which so gradu-"ally liquefies and swells that the change which it is under-"going is only recognized when after some time it becomes "softened and expanded.

"*Sensible* fermentation is the adventitious * * * * * *
"bodies themselves and is recognized by the senses so soon as
"ever it begins. Such is the fermentation which is brought
"about when water is poured on quick-lime, or spirits of
"vitriol is mixed with oil of tartar.

   "*Vehement* fermentation is the adventitious * * * * * *
"sensible cause, which quickly brings about an essential
"change or a conspicuous alteration in the fermenting bodies
"themselves and is produced with a certain impetus and
"indeed sometimes with considerable tumult. Of this kind
"is the movement which is observed when spirits of vitriol
"is poured on oil of tartar or water on quick-lime.

   "*Moderate* fermentation is the adventitious * * * * * *
"which brings about an essential change or a conspicuous
"alteration in the fermenting bodies themselves gradually and
"without a rush, and with a certain buzzing only (fremitus) or
"without any noise or buzzing.

   "Of this kind is that movement which must or wort, as
"for instance that of beer, treacle and things of that kind,
"undergoes when it ferments, and which takes place with a
"certain buzzing.

   "*Hot* fermentation which properly and deservedly gains the
"name of fermentation is the adventitious * * * * * * in the
"fermenting bodies themselves, and is accompanied by or
"quickly acquires heat. Such is that which is observed when
"vinegar is mixed with quick-lime, which indeed is accom-
"panied with fire and flame and therefore heat.

   "*Cold* fermentation is the * * * * * * and is produced
"without any heat. Of this kind is that when coral is dis-
"solved in vinegar."

   This confusion of fermentation, properly so called, with the
effervescence due to the escape of gas from simple direct
chemical action, though undoubtedly a retrograde step, may
be regarded with leniency when we reflect that it was only one
of many indications of the special attitude of Sylvius's mind,
through which, though he went too far, he did good service by
shewing that the importance and pertinency to physiology of
van Helmont's chemical views might be recognized without
accepting his spiritualistic speculations.

Sylvius followed van Helmont in so far as the latter insisted that many of the phenomena of the living body were to be explained by the help of chemical science as the outcome of chemical processes, a view which physiologists had before van Helmont too much neglected; but he refused to follow him in regarding chemical changes as mere instruments in the hands of occult spiritual agencies. On the contrary he boldly asserted that the chemistry of living things was the same as the chemistry of so-called dead things, that what took place in a live body was the same as that which might be made to take place in a flask in the laboratory. And filled as his mind was with the striking results which he had obtained in the laboratory as he worked with salts, with acids, and with bases, he jumped to the conclusion that the chemistry of the living body was of the same order, and that an adequate knowledge of acids and alkalis was the key to the interpretation of the problems of life.

In taking up this position he performed at least one useful task, he brought the chemical investigation of physiological problems into line with the mechanical and physical investigation of them. The spiritualistic fancies of van Helmont, and still more the earlier ones of Paracelsus, had had the tendency to make men think that chemical inquiry in contrast with physical inquiry was in some way necessarily bound up with speculations about invisible agencies of a spiritual kind; and this doubtless was more or less a bar to men of sober and exact thought entering upon that line of inquiry. To Sylvius at least is due the credit of shewing that there was no such necessary connection between chemistry and spiritualism; that on the contrary the newer chemistry in its attempts to solve vital problems trod the path of the most naked materialism. It is probably to his thus opening up a line of inquiry into chemical physiology free from all taint of mysticism that the great influence which as a teacher he undoubtedly exercised was largely due.

Sylvius had the advantage over van Helmont of the knowledge of three important discoveries which were not made until after the latter's death. Van Helmont knew only of the gastric juice, the acid ferment of the stomach, and of bile as digestive juices; for we may omit his stercoraceous ferment of the caecum. Sylvius knew of others. We have already seen that in 1655 and 1661 Wharton and Stensen discovered the submaxillary and parotid ducts. On the importance of these two discoveries with reference to the physiology of secretion I have already spoken; they were still more important as regards digestion. Stensen paid little attention, and Wharton hardly any at all to the digestive uses of saliva; but Sylvius seized at once on its importance, and as we shall see attributed to it very large powers.

He was also through the investigations of a pupil of his led to recognize the possibly great uses of another digestive juice. Wirsung had, we have seen, discovered in 1642 the pancreatic duct, and appears to have observed the pancreatic juice; but he did not pursue the subject, and indeed his discovery remained barren until one of Sylvius' scholars took the matter up. The work of the latter is so interesting an example of the physiological experiments of the time that I venture to speak of it in some detail.

Regnier de Graaf, born in 1641 at Schoonhoven in Holland, of a good family, studied under Sylvius at Leyden, and after graduating and travelling, practised for some years at Delft, where he died in 1673 at the early age of 32, having in the previous year refused to succeed to the Chair at Leyden, just vacant by the death of his late master Sylvius. While at Delft he published some remarkable works on the structure of the generative organs, and described the follicles in the ovary which have ever since been known by his name. It was however while a student at Leyden under Sylvius, in 1664, as yet a youth of 23, that he made an investigation on pancreatic juice, published under the title of *Disputatio medica de natura et usu succi pancreatici.*

In this tract after relating several unsuccessful attempts by various methods at obtaining the juice he tells us how he hit upon the right one. He made use of the quill of a wild duck, which he says may be got longer and thinner than the quill of any other bird. Into the far, narrower end of this he inserted a plug of soft wood, attached to which, and carried through the quill, was a long thread, by which the plug could be withdrawn. Having performed tracheotomy on a dog (and he recommends that the animal should be fasting) he opened the abdomen, ligatured the duodenum below the pylorus, and below the entrance of the bile and pancreatic ducts, laid open the duodenum, sponged the interior carefully, and then introduced the quill into the mouth of the duct. The near, broader end of the quill was, by means of rolls of paper smeared with paste, firmly fitted into the neck of a small flask, in the body of which was an orifice made on purpose to allow air to escape, and through which the thread attached to the plug of the quill was drawn. By the help of rings round the neck of the flask it and the quill were securely fastened in their place, and the wound in the abdomen, from which the flask hung down, carefully sewn up. By means of the thread the plug in the quill was then withdrawn and in a short time the juice was observed to drop into the flask. In this way De Graaf succeeded in obtaining from two drachms to half an ounce, and in one case, that of a large dog, a whole ounce of juice, in some seven or eight hours.

This first cannalisation of the pancreatic duct seems to have been adopted as a temporary measure only; there is no statement of the animal having been kept alive for any length of time. By the same method De Graaf also obtained saliva from the parotid duct, and bile from the bile duct. He collected parotid saliva and pancreatic juice from the same animal at the same time, and observed that the two juices differed in their characters. It is interesting to note that this experiment on the pancreas was never, so far as is known, repeated by anyone until Claude Bernard in modern times took it up again.

De Graaf's record of the examination of the qualities or characters of the juice is very meagre. There is no account of any distinct chemical examination, he chiefly tested it by the sense of taste. And he states that thus tested its qualities were found to vary; it was sometimes insipid, at other times acid or rough, often salt, but most frequently acid-salt.

He records that he had an opportunity once of examining the pancreatic juice of a sailor who had died quite suddenly, and that he found the human juice identical in its properties with that of the dog.

De Graaf then goes on to discuss the uses of this pancreatic juice in digestion, and what he says may be taken as part of the general teaching of Sylvius concerning digestion.

Van Helmont, knowing nothing of either salivary or pancreatic ducts, held, as we have seen, that digestion consists wholly in the two actions of the acid ferment of the stomach and of the ferment of the bile. Sylvius on the contrary (naturally perhaps inclined to give too much weight to a new discovery) was led to attach the greatest possible importance to saliva; he regarded it as the type of fermentative juices, of what he calls a mild character, and attributed much of the changes taking place in the stomach to the saliva swallowed with the food rather than to the ferment provided by the stomach itself. He appears to have considered that the mucus (pituita as it was called) clinging to the interior of the intestine was in reality the remains of the swallowed saliva; and he went so far as to hint that the change which the blood undergoes in the lungs may be due to a mingling of the venous blood of the pulmonary artery with some fluid secreted by the trachea and bronchi, or with the saliva which somehow or other found its way to the lungs.

It was saliva then, in Sylvius's opinion, which was the chief agent in bringing about the first stage of the fermentation called chylification. The second stage, according to him, is due to interaction of the bile and pancreatic juice. We have seen that De Graaf tried to persuade himself, by taste chiefly, that the pancreatic juice was acid, and indeed the acidity of the pancreatic juice was a foundation-stone of Sylvius's views on digestion. Although, as we have seen, his chemical inquiries were chiefly concerned with acids, alkalis and bases, and he was above all other men of his time qualified to speak about such things, although he might have been expected to be one of the first to recognize that pancreatic juice was alkaline, he nevertheless, led away apparently by preconceived theory, always insisted that it was acid. Its use in digestion was, he said, and De Graaf repeated it, to effervesce, to ferment, with the bile. Sylvius says:

"It is impossible that the juice of the pancreas in some "degree or mode so acid should be mixed with the bile,

"abounding as this does in bitter and volatile salt, without
"exciting an effervescence, as may be proved by endless ex-
"amples seen in chemistry and elsewhere."

So also De Graaf: "That effervescence is excited by the
"mixture of pancreatic juice which abounds in acidity, with
"bile which abounds in volatile and fixed salt, we dare all the
"more boldly assert, since hitherto we have met with no
"example of an acid spirit meeting with a lixivious salt (*i.e.*
"a soluble salt derived by washing ashes) without a manifest
"effervescence resulting, provided impediments are removed."

De Graaf recognized the difficulty presented by the fact
that when bile and pancreatic juice are mixed together out
of the body they do not effervesce; but he overcomes this
by arguing that in this as in so many other cases a suitable
temperature is needed. "However it be, no one ought to
"wonder that we cannot demonstrate an effervescence be-
"tween bile and pancreatic juice when these are mixed
"together outside the living body, since neither artificial heat
"nor the natural warmth of the hand can excite such a heat
"as we know exists in the small intestine on account of the
"surroundings of the very warm viscera."

He also notices the objection that the dilution of the mixed
juices with the chyle would interfere with the effervescence;
but he argues that dilution may favour effervescence. "We
"answer," says he, "that oil of vitriol mixed with water ex-
"cites a far more violent effervescence with iron filings than
"when it is used pure without any water." So completely did
Sylvius and his school identify physiological fermentation
with chemical effervescence.

Confident as Sylvius and his pupil were of the occurrence
and of the importance of this effervescence of pancreatic juice
and bile, they were far from clear as to how it promoted
digestion. De Graaf gives two uses. The effervescence in the
first place attenuates the viscid mucus lining the interior of
the intestine, the presence of which might hinder the absorption of chyle by the lacteals; and in the second place it assists
the due separation of the useful parts of the food from the
useless. But he does not explain how it does this. It is interesting to note that he attributes the white colour observable

in the duodenum beyond the entrance of the pancreatic
duct to the pancreatic juice. "As regards," says he, "the
"whitish colour observable in the more fluid parts of the food,
"we think that is due to the acidity of the pancreatic juice,
"for we have observed that many other things abounding
"in lixivious (soluble) salt and oil whiten upon the addition
"of acids." Here again we see how completely the school of
Sylvius identified physiological changes with changes of a
purely chemical nature.

In the time of Sylvius men's minds were full of the discovery
of the lacteals, the thoracic duct and the lymphatics, and Sylvius
had no manner of doubt that all the chyle, that is to say,
all the nutritious parts of the food, passed into the lacteals and
were so discharged into the venous system through the thoracic
duct. The blood carried to the right side of the heart by the
upper great veins was in his view chylous blood. In the right
side of the heart it met with the blood of the vena cava, and
this Sylvius speaks of as bilious blood. Following the idea
which van Helmont seems to have held that bile is secreted
by the gall-bladder, Sylvius warmly espoused a view which
had been recently put forward, that that part of the bile
which was not needed for digestion was carried back to the
liver, where it passed into the venous system and whence,
mixed with the blood, it was carried by the vena cava to the
heart. This erroneous view (a retrograde step from the position
taken up by Vesalius) was disproved by Glisson, and later on,
as we have seen, more distinctly by Malpighi; but Sylvius
long clung to it. It fitted into his general theory. "Chyle,"
he says, "assumes the form of blood (a superficial initial
"change) owing to the bilious blood ascending to the heart
"meeting in the right auricle and especially in the right
"ventricle with the lymphatic blood (of the superior vena
"cava) with which the chyle is mixed, and so on account of
"the different or rather opposite disposition of each (kind of
"blood) in certain of their parts provoking an effervescence
"of great moment." This is the initial change on the right
side of the heart; but "the chyle reaches (not the superficial
"form only, but) the ultimate perfection of blood through
"the continued and tempered effervescence, presently to be

"described, which by reason of the breathing of air takes place
"in the lungs, in the left auricle and ventricle of the heart,
"and in the large trunks of the aorta. By the energy and help
"of this effervescence we think that there bursts out and
"springs forth the vital fire (ignis vitalis), which by rarefying
"the more fatty and oily parts, not only of the chyle added
"to the blood, but of the blood itself, and by loosely uniting
"together at the same time all other parts, reduces the whole
"into a heterogeneous, homogeneous mass, and so converts
"the chyle into true blood."

All this is wordy and vague enough; nor is he at all more
distinct when he dwells on that breathing of air which, as he
has just said, brings abôut the above changes. After giving a
fair description of the mechanics of respiration he goes on to
say:

"By what power, however, or in what manner and way the
"inspired air so alters the blood is not equally clear. I, for my
"part, think that it is brought about by reason of there being
"dispersed in the air nitrous and subacid particles able to
"condense the rarefied and boiling blood and so to gently
"restrain its ebullition."

Wordy and vague as his exposition is, we cannot however
fail to recognize the efforts of a man working on van Helmont's
lines, but attempting to shew that the fuller knowledge of
chemical change which he had gained by studying the actions
and reactions of various liquids and salts, which now dissolving, now precipitating each other, now provoking, now
checking ebullition or effervescence, that is to say the
development of gas, pointed to the conclusion that it was
unnecessary to take refuge in subtle influences and occult
agencies, but that all the changes in the body were but larger
and more complex examples of the changes which could be
produced in the laboratory.

This is pointedly shewn by what Sylvius taught concerning
the secretion of urine. I have already referred to Borelli's
mechanical theory of renal secretion. Sylvius is not content
with this. He says:

"Although one may reasonably suspect that the material
"of the urine undergoes some special change while it is being

"strained through the papillae of the kidneys, it seems to me
"exceedingly probable at least that the blood and even the
"chyle is in the heart itself, through the vital effervescence
"which it there undergoes, prepared for the secretion of the
"urinary serosity, and that it is the completion only of the
"secretion which takes place in the kidneys." And then follow
these remarkable words: "Although I cannot as yet fully
"follow out the process, nevertheless I hope to arrive at it by
"the process of precipitation."

Reading between the lines by the help of the knowledge
which we have gained since those days, we may find in Sylvius's
words a prophecy of that limitation, in which we now believe,
of the work of the kidney to the task of secreting, by mere
elimination, the urea already formed in the tissues and carried
to the kidney by the blood. But I quote the words also to
shew how complete was Sylvius's confidence in his chemical
methods. The change in the blood preparatory to the actual
work of the kidney itself, was, he had no doubt, a mere
chemical process, such as he might imitate in his laboratory,
adding one clear liquid to another, and observing how a
cloud of solid particles made its appearance, particles which
might be strained off by a sieve such as the kidney seemed
to be.

Borelli, as we have seen, while accepting the old view of
animal spirits residing in the brain and nerves, framed a
physical mechanical conception of them; in his eyes the
animal spirits became a fluid of peculiar physical features,
but still a corporeal fluid, acting in a mechanical way. Sylvius
also accepts the animal spirits, but to him they become a
chemical fluid, a fluid with chemical properties, a fluid of the
type of common alcohol, existing, flowing in a pure state
perhaps in the nerves, but capable of mixing elsewhere with
the blood. This is seen in his view of the spleen:

"Since the spleen serves neither for sensation nor mere
"movement, it must be for some other purpose that it receives
"in such notable quantities the animal spirits (as indicated by
"its great nerve supply). For what end can it receive these
"except that they may enter into and be intimately mixed
"with the inflowing (arterial) blood, and make that blood

"more subtle and spirituous than its wont, that is to say,
"more complete than the rest of the (arterial) blood which is
"already perfect, in other words, more than perfect?"

These two men, Borelli and Sylvius, stand out in the middle
of the seventeenth century as the founders of two distinct,
and indeed contending schools of thought. Borelli sought to
explain most, if not all, of the phenomena of the living body as
mere problems of the new mathematical, mechanical, physical
science, and so became the founder of the iatro-mathematical
school. Sylvius sought to explain the same phenomena as
mere problems of the newborn chemical science, and so
became the founder of the iatro-chemical school. But the
two were men of a very different mould.

Borelli had a foundation of exact, definite, proved knowledge to build upon; his mind was a strong and acute one;
he himself rarely, if ever, went further than facts and his
reason led him, save perhaps when he, as all his school are
tempted to do, trusted too much to the power of a formula
to carry him over gaps where a knowledge of facts was
wanting. He would have been the first to scoff at the handiwork of some coming after him who called themselves his
disciples.

Sylvius had no such exact knowledge at his back. He was
groping his way in the dim twilight of a rising but not yet
risen science; in that dim light he confounded shadows with
things, and mistook the size of images looming in the mist of
the dawn.

Moreover, he had neither the strength nor the width of
mind of Borelli. He was one of those who think that a well-
sounding phrase is of necessity a carrier of truth, and he was
also one of those who are prepared to explain everything,
and are satisfied themselves with every explanation which
they give. For almost every physiological problem he had a
chemical illustration ready at hand; and he seems to have had
no manner of doubt that an adequate knowledge of alkalis
and acids would carry him triumphantly through all the difficulties both of health and disease. While Borelli was in the
main a philosopher only, Sylvius was an active physician;
as he considered health to be ordered and appropriate

chemical change, so he regarded disease to be excessive or deficient or perverted chemical change, a change which he hoped to cure by the skilful addition or withdrawal of acids and the like. And though his followers abused chemical, as much as Borelli's followers abused physical, knowledge, none of them perhaps ever exceeded their master in the unbounded confidence which he had in the validity of his method.

The importance of Sylvius in the history of physiology attaches, as we have seen, rather to his zealous teaching of the value of chemical knowledge as a means of solving vital problems, than to any special discoveries of his own. He was happier when dealing with digestion than with other phenomena, though his success in this he owed largely to Stensen and De Graaf. And one cannot but admit that in attaching such great importance as he did to the pancreatic juice, wrong as his interpretation of the nature of the action of that juice might have been, he anticipated by some two centuries the labours of Claude Bernard. But even that merit soon seemed to be taken away from him.

In the year 1653, just as Sylvius was rising into note, there was born at Schaffhausen in Switzerland one Jean Conrad Peyer, who, studying at Basel and Paris, practised in his native town, dying there in 1712.

In 1677, five years after Sylvius's death, Peyer published a little tract, *Exercitatio anatomica medica de glandulis intestinorum*, in which he described certain new glands, scattered over the intestine, which he says he had discovered in 1673. In this work he gives a very careful account of the bodies ever since known by his name, indicating their position on the free border of the intestine, and their increased abundance in the lower part of the small intestine, in the ileum, and distinguishing between the single solitary glands and the patches of agminated glands. He describes them however as being provided, each, with a minute pore opening into the interior of the intestine, through which when the gland is pressed a pale fluid exudes. He discusses at some length whether the new glands are conglomerate (secretory) in nature, or conglobate (lymphatic), and decides in favour of the former view on the grounds that each gland possesses

a duct, and is well supplied with arteries, whereas no lacteals
or lymphatics seem to proceed from it, and indeed the lacteals
arise from the attached border of the intestine, whereas the
glands in question are found on the free border.

He argues that the secretion from these glands must play
an important part in the digestion of food, and suggests that
they are more abundant in the lower part of the intestine
because as the food descends from the duodenum the efficacy
of the pancreatic juice must become more and more exhausted.

This discovery by Peyer fitted in very well with another
discovery made a few years later by another Jean Conrad.
Jean Conrad von Brunner, born at Dieffenhofen in 1653, the
same year as Peyer, after studying and graduating at Strassburg, and travelling in Holland, France, and England, was in
1687 called to the Chair of Medicine in Heidelberg. He afterwards became Court physician at Düsseldorf, and having had
great success in practice died at Mannheim in 1727.

In 1682, five years before his call to Heidelberg, he published a little work, *Experimenta nova circa pancreas*, embodying the results of work which he had begun ten years before.

In this he made known that he had succeeded several times
in removing from a dog nearly the whole of the pancreas, and
in keeping the animal alive afterwards for a considerable time.
He removed nearly, but not quite, the whole of the gland; the
extreme end lay so deep in the body that it could not be
reached by the knife.

He insisted that the animal when it recovered from the
effects of the operation, as in most cases it did, in no way
suffered in health. It ate, drank, ran about as usual, was
well-nourished, and all its digestive functions were carried on
normally. Obviously, says Brunner, Sylvius and De Graaf
were wholly wrong in attributing the importance which they
did to the digestive powers of the pancreatic juice. The
animals on which I operated secreted no pancreatic juice into
the intestine, the duct and nearly the whole gland having
been done away with; yet they digested as usual.

Upon entering into the professorial chair at Heidelberg, in
1687, Brunner published a *Dissertatio inauguralis de glandulis*

duodeni, in which he described the glands since known by his name. He states that these glands yield a fluid like pancreatic juice, and he speaks of them as being a 'pancreas secundarium.' He had mentioned his results of extirpation of the pancreas to his friend Peyer before the latter wrote the tract just mentioned; and Peyer saw in Brunner's experiments a confirmation of his view that the glands described by him carried out an important part of intestinal digestion. Brunner himself however was inclined to think that Peyer's glands only secreted a mere mucosity, and that the really active agent in intestinal digestion was to be found in Brunner's glands.

In view of the connection between extirpation of the pancreas and glycosuria made known by modern researches it may be interesting to note that in an experiment in which Brunner had first removed the spleen, and on recovery from that operation the pancreas also, "it was especially to be seen "that the animal made water very frequently, and that he "was very thirsty, drinking largely of water in proportion to "the discharge of urine." But as Brunner observes, the acute Malpighi has noticed a similar result after ligature of the vessels of the spleen only. These are Malpighi's words:

"In a dog of as yet tender years a wound was made in the "left hypochondrium, and the blood vessels of the protruding "spleen and attached omentum were ligatured with a thread "close to the hilus of the spleen; everything was presently "replaced in its former position, the peritoneum and the "muscles were sutured and the skin loosely united. After the "lapse of a few days the wound had healed. After some weeks "the animal was strong enough to perform with enjoyment "all its proper functions; so long as it lived no trace of any "interference with health could be observed. Having become "more hungry than before, it took its meals eagerly, devouring "bones and food of all kinds. One thing only I observed, "namely that it made water abundantly and most frequently, "in fact continually. Though all dogs are continually doing "this, it seemed in this respect to outdo all its fellows. Its "habit of body was in every respect sound; indeed it became "fat, and in other respects, in quickness and alacrity, it "equalled its fellows."

Post-mortem examination shewed an atrophy of the spleen, but hardly any other abnormality.

In another experiment, in which the pancreas alone was removed, Brunner observes: "I had bought the animal from "a butcher, and after the operation it also was hungry. It "was continually going to its old master's shop and stealing "pieces of meat. Indeed it carried on this game to such an "extent that the butcher came to me and demanded that it "should be killed. This however I put off doing since I "wanted to enjoy for some time longer such a pleasant "experience as the animal's condition afforded me." In another experiment too the animal was particularly hungry and greedy; but in this case it is especially noted that there was no other symptom, "he was not more thirsty than before "the operation."

With Brunner and Peyer's discovery, the short-lived glory of the pancreatic juice, raised up for it by Sylvius and De Graaf, passed away. The minds of physiologists went back to the older view that the stomach was the chief seat of digestion, and that bile either served in some way as an aid to gastric digestion, or was merely an excrement.

Concerning gastric digestion itself, two views contended for prominence. Borelli, with his mind directed chiefly to mechanical effects, had pointed out the great grinding, crushing force which was provided for by the muscular coats of the stomach. He calls attention to the fact "that in birds, with "few exceptions, the crushing, erosion and trituration of food "is effected by the muscular stomach itself, compressing one "part of its horny lining against another. Thus with the help "of small hard and sharp pebbles contained in it, which serve "instead of teeth, the stomach by pounding the food swallowed "and rubbing its inner surfaces on it this way and that, like "millstones, crushes the parts of the food until they are con-"verted into a very fine powder. This at Pisa, at the bidding "of His Serene Highness Duke Ferdinand II, I ascertained by "experiment to be quite true. For I introduced by the mouth "into the stomach of turkeys glass globules, or empty "vesicles, and leaden cubes, similarly hollowed out, pyramids of "wood and many other things, and the next day I found the

"leaden masses crushed and eroded, the glass pulverized and
"the remaining ingesta in the same condition."

He admits however that birds of prey and fishes which are
destitute of teeth and possess not a fleshy but a membranous
stomach like that of a quadruped, digest their hard food in
a different manner. "These animals consume flesh and bones
"by means of a certain very potent ferment much in the same
"way as corrosive liquids corrode and dissolve metals. Such a
"corrosive juice is poured forth by the small glands with which
"the membranous substance of the stomach is crowded, as
"I have most clearly seen in the stomach of the Dolphin, in
"which the small glands are very stout and prominent."

Quantitative as he always was he desired to estimate the
exact force of these muscles of the stomach, and he proceeded
on the same plan as that which he had adopted for determining
the force of the heart systole.

"Having noticed that some filberts possess a shell so hard
"that they can hardly be broken by the molar teeth of man,
"I introduced some of these by the mouth into the stomachs
"of turkeys and observed on the following day that they were
"broken and pulverized. And because it might be supposed
"that their woody husks had been macerated and softened by
"some fermentative juice, I forthwith introduced into the
"stomachs of other turkeys glass vesicles, so stout that they
"could with difficulty be crushed with the teeth, and I found
"these on the following day in the faeces reduced to powder.

"Hence since the action of these two organs, that is to say,
"the teeth and the fleshy stomach, is similar, for they act by
"pressure like a winepress, and overcome the same resistance,
"viz. the hardness of the same glass vesicles, we may therefore
"conclude that the motive powers of the two are equal. But
"we have already shewn that the absolute force of the muscles
"which close the human jaw represents a power greater than
"that of a weight of 1350 lbs. Therefore the force of the
"turkey's stomach is not less than the power of 1350 lbs."

Borelli, as we have just seen, though he appears to think
that in most birds the digestive action is wholly mechanical,
and indeed he maintained that the pebbles in the stomach
might be not only mere mechanical aids, but when crushed

might serve for nutriment, admits in the case of some stomachs a corrosive juice. In this point as in others the followers of Borelli went beyond their master, and the iatro-physical school after him were prepared to deny chemical action in all cases, and to maintain that digestion was in reality a mere trituration of the food by the muscular mill of the stomach into the creamy mass known as chyle.

The iatro-chemical school on the one hand, following van Helmont and Sylvius, contended that the change in the stomach was chiefly if not wholly a chemical change effected by a process of fermentation. Opinions differed however as to what was the efficient agent of the process. It was generally recognized that the lining membrane of the stomach was glandular in nature; this in many creatures, such as birds, was obvious. But many were inclined to attach greater im-portance to a juice, such as the saliva, which was poured forth by a conspicuous duct, than to a fluid which seemed simply to ooze from a membranous surface; and these were led to regard the change in the stomach as brought about not by the independent action of a ferment belonging, as van Helmont had thought, to the stomach itself, but by such a ferment with the help of the swallowed saliva, or even by the saliva itself.

After the works which I have just mentioned we have to wait a long time, for many years, for in fact the greater part of a century, before we come upon another solid addition to our knowledge of the subject.

It is true that during the remainder of the seventeenth century new truths about chemistry, new views about chemical action were being continually gathered in. It is true that at the close of the seventeenth and the beginning of the eighteenth century there flourished two men who achieved great eminence as chemists and who were assiduous in apply-ing their chemical knowledge to physiology; but so far at least as digestion is concerned their influence was that rather of expositors than of discoverers. One of these was George Ernest Stahl, who was born at Anspach in 1660 at the time when Sylvius was in his fullest vigour. After studying and graduating at Jena, he became Court physician at Weimar, and in 1694 Professor of Medicine at Halle; but in 1716, being made physician to the King of Prussia, he moved to Berlin, where he died in 1734. He was an accomplished chemist, and his name must always be borne in mind in dealing with the history of science, if for nothing else for the reason that he was the author of the famous theory of phlogiston, which ruled with a rod of iron, as it were, the thoughts of natural philosophers for a hundred years.

His general views he seems to have learnt, in the first instance, from Wedel, his teacher at Jena, who was an ardent spiritualist and who wrote a tract on the archaeus; but in chemistry he sat at the feet of Johann Joachim Beccher, of whose *Physica Subterranea*, a treatise on chemistry, he published an edition in 1703. Beccher developed at some length his views on the essential principle of fire, but does not seem to have used the word phlogiston. In the *Specimen Beccherianum* which Sylvius appended to his edition of the *Physica*, and in which he expounds Beccher's theoretical views, he says, "Briefly, in the act of composition, as an instrument "there intervenes and is most potent, fire, flaming, fervid, "hot; but in the very substance of the compound there in-"tervenes, as an ingredient, as it is commonly called, as a "material principle and as a constituent part of the whole "compound the material and principle of fire, not fire itself. "This I was the first to call phlogiston." He had used the phrase several years before, as early as 1697 at least.

The pendulum swung far in one direction when Sylvius threw aside all van Helmont's subtleties and spiritualistic conceptions, his ferments which acted with a power higher than and different from that governing ordinary chemical changes, his archaei of which the ferments were the instruments, and his sensitive soul of which the archaei were the servants—threw aside I say all these and maintained that the events of the living body were ordinary chemical events, and attempted to explain digestion, respiration, and everything else by means of an effervescence like that which he witnessed when vitriol was thrown on iron filings or on long-exposed ashes. But the pendulum swung back again in the

old direction, with as great if not greater impetus when Stahl
put forward and brilliantly maintained the view that all the
chemical events of the living body, even though they might
superficially resemble, were at the bottom wholly different
from the chemical changes taking place in the laboratory,
since in the living body all chemical changes were directly
governed by the sensitive soul, *anima sensitiva*, which per-
vaded all parts and presided over all events.

Stahl's 'sensitive soul,' of which I shall have somewhat
more to say in a subsequent Lecture, was something very
different both from the sensitive soul of van Helmont and
the rational soul of Descartes. To the latter indeed it was,
in truth, in full antagonism. In Descartes' view, the human
body apart from the rational soul was a machine, and the
phenomena of man, apart from those which were the direct
expression of the activity of the rational soul, were the
phenomena of a machine governed by ordinary physical laws;
had chemistry been as advanced in Descartes' time as in
Stahl's he might have added chemical laws. To Stahl, on the
contrary, a machine was exactly that which the animal body
was not; its phenomena were not the phenomena governed
by physical and chemical laws, but phenomena obeying laws
of a wholly different kind, the laws of the sensitive soul; the
sensitive soul made itself felt in even the simplest and so to
say lowest changes of the body.

With van Helmont, Stahl had much more kinship, and
indeed his views may to a certain extent be regarded as a
development of van Helmont's; the sensitive soul of Stahl is
that of van Helmont with two differences only. The sensitive
soul of Stahl works directly on chemical processes, withou
the intervention of archaei, and is not a mortal something
associated with, and as it were the shell of, an immortal mind,
but it is itself the immortal principle, spiritual and immaterial,
coming from afar, and at the death of the body returning to
whence it came.

Stahl's fundamental position is that between living things,
so long as they are alive, however simple, and non-living
things, however composite, however complex in their phenomena, there is a great gulf fixed. The former, so long as they

are alive, are actuated by an immaterial agent, the sensitive soul, the latter are not. This position he develops at great length in his treatise, *De mixti et vivi corporis vera diversitate,* 'On the real difference between a chemical compound and a living body.'

A living body is distinguished from a non-living merely compound body by the fact that though capable of change and indeed, in the very development of its activity, continually undergoing changes, it nevertheless maintains for a given period an identical existence.

"This very preservation of a thing essentially destructible "by which its destruction through its own activity is pre- "vented is exactly that which we ought to understand by the "common word 'vital.' This is the feature by the absence of "which a body so far as it is simply a compound body con- "trasts with and is distinguished from a body which is living."

Further, the living body is fitted for special ends and purposes; the living body does not exist for itself; it is con- stituted to be the true and continued minister of the soul. The body is made for the soul, the soul is not made for, and is not the product of, the body.

"We may therefore rightly and truly conclude that all the "actions of the body, both those which concern its structure "and those which relate to the preservation of its composition, "are carried out by the soul itself for its own uses and ends, "and are directed and brought to completion, knowingly and "properly, in the proportions and relations which fit those "ends and uses."

The soul builds up the body and makes use of it for its own ends:

"Vital activities are directly administered and exercised "by the soul itself, and are truly organic acts carried out in "corporeal instruments by a superior acting cause, in order to "bring about certain effects, which are not only in general "certain, and in particular necessary, but also in each and "every particular adapted, in a special and yet most com- "plete manner, to the needs of the moment and to the "various irregularities introduced by accidental external "causes. Vital activities, vital movements, cannot, as some

"recent crude speculations suppose, have any real likeness
"to such movements as, in an ordinary way, depend on the
"material condition of a body and take place without any
"direct use or end or aim."

Van Helmont, as we have seen, regarded archaei in the first
degree, and ferments in the second, as agents intervening
between matter, with its material properties, and the immaterial sensitive soul. Stahl ridicules the idea of there being
any need of a number of such intermediate agencies between
the soul and matter. One link between spirit and matter is
necessary, and one only: that one is 'motion.'

"That which both preserves the whole body and provides
"for and carries out the uses of the soul in the body is a
"something which on the one hand is quite different from the
"essential and proper nature of the body itself, and on the
"other hand is twin to the essential, absolute and genuine
"nature of the soul itself—a something which is in itself
"incorporeal, just like the soul itself, but powerful and active
"in the actual body, like again the soul itself. Moreover,
"it is clear that this something ministers to the wants of
"the soul, not only so far as the existence and maintenance
"of the body is concerned, but also and especially in the naked,
"pure, and direct uses and purposes of the soul. And that in
"such a way that the soul even in its highest functions and
"in its supreme activity has such clear, true, full power over
"this something of which we are speaking, that it quite
"absolutely governs it, increases it, diminishes it, and turns
"or directs it, according to its judgment. This something
"indeed so simply and absolutely belongs to the soul, even
"in its most direct acts, that whenever anything which is
"truly and essentially belonging to a part of the soul sets out
"to become active, or to accomplish anything, it always
"discharges that duty, always accomplishes that act by means
"of this very something of which I am speaking, which thus
"serves as its true instrument; this something, however, is
"nothing else than 'motion.' By motion indeed the soul
"carries out all its doings."

And he goes on to shew how all the phenomena of the living
body, in their threefold aspects, the phenomena concerned

in the preservation of the material composition of the body, in the formation and repair of structures, and in sensation with all its consequences, are all of them, to use the words of a modern writer, at bottom 'modes of motion.'

Stahl applies these views to the physiology of digestion. He admits, or seems to admit, fermentation as a property of non-living things, and seems to regard putrefaction as a sort of fermentation also possible in and belonging to non-living things. He even seems to admit that the ferments of saliva and pancreatic juice are such non-living agencies; though he refuses to believe in a gastric ferment. "Some people suppose "that gastric digestion results from the action of particular "and specific ferments, and indeed go so far as to regard the "stomach as not only the seat but also the origin of a par- "ticular ferment, whereas in the whole construction of the "stomach nothing peculiar is observed which would render "the elaboration of such a special agent likely."

But even admitting the existence and action of various ferments, the physiology of digestion is according to Stahl still far from being explained.

"Although the medical schools, following van Helmont, "rightly judge, as a general conclusion, that the resolution "of food takes place after the fashion of a fermentation, the "particular way in which it occurs is involved in almost in- "superable difficulties. The chief of these consists in this that "not only the fermentation of fermentable things takes place 'far more rapidly in the stomach than outside it, but also, "things subject outside the body to no fermentation at all, "unless it be that of putrefaction, undergo as it were a special "kind of fermentation in the stomach, and do not follow that "kind to which under other circumstances they are prone, but "are overtaken and overcome by this digestive fermentation. "Then there is the specific character which is imposed on the "digested material as is seen in the differences which exist in "even the crude chyle, or the milk of different animals living "on exactly the same food.

"In any case the fermentation which takes place in the "alimentary canal is not an ordinary fermentation such as "occurs in a merely compound non-living body, but a most "special character is impressed on the change, impressed by "the energy of the soul."

Stahl's teaching, in fact, was briefly this:

Learn as much as you can of chemical and physical processes, and in so far as the phenomena of the living body exactly resemble chemical and physical events occurring in non-living bodies, you may explain them by chemical and physical laws. But do not conclude that that which you see taking place in a non-living body will take place in a living body, for the chemical and physical phenomena of the latter are modified by the soul. The events of the body may be rough hewn by chemical and physical forces, but the soul will shape them to its own ends, and will do that by its instrument, motion.

He thus stands forth at the close of the seventeenth century as the founder of 'animism,' which doctrine, though his sensitive soul fell back later to the lower stage of 'a vital principle,' maintained itself in many minds through the two succeeding centuries, and exists at the present day.

The other man, a man of a wholly different mind, was Hermann Boerhaave; but of him it will be best to speak in connection with his even more illustrious pupil Albrecht von Haller, and in this aspect he belongs wholly to the eighteenth century.

LECTURE VII

THE ENGLISH SCHOOL OF THE SEVENTEENTH CENTURY. THE PHYSIOLOGY OF RESPIRATION

WHILE we have been following the gradual enlightenment of the physiological world we have seen how the spot of light which was the centre of illumination shifted from place to place, and shone now in one University, now in another. We have seen it bursting out brilliantly at Padua in Vesalius, less brightly in Fabricius; it appeared meteor-like in Switzerland in Paracelsus; then it moved to London and shone in Harvey. Anon it burst out in the Northern countries in van Helmont at Brussels, in Stensen at Copenhagen. It flitted back to Italy, to Borelli in Pisa, to Malpighi in Bologna, and once more returned to the North to Sylvius in Leyden and to others.

I have now to ask you to go back with me once more to London. Englishmen are justly proud of Harvey, and they take some credit for Glisson. They may also boast of a little band, worthy successors of Harvey, who in the middle and latter part of the seventeenth century made remarkable progress in the knowledge of the true nature of breathing.

The exact physical science which Galileo had begun at Pisa soon crossed the seas and passed to England, stirring up a knot of men to pursue studies of the same kind, a knot of men who some few years afterwards founded the Royal Society of London, for the advancement of natural knowledge, in the hope, a hope not wholly unfulfilled, that it would help them in their "attempts by actual experiments to shape out "a new philosophy or to perfect the old."

Conspicuous among these was a gentleman of leisure, of noble birth, the Honourable Robert Boyle, whose keen intellect pierced far into every problem to which he turned his mind, and who touched nothing without leaving his mark upon it.

It would be out of place for me here to attempt to give even a sketch of Boyle's influence on the progress of physical and chemical science. I must content myself with speaking only of his notable contribution to the solution of respiratory problems, a contribution which was part of and incidental to his researches on the general properties of the atmosphere.

Before doing so I must briefly recall to your minds the progress which had been made in the knowledge of this subject of respiration up to the time when Boyle made his notable experiment.

In the old Galenic doctrine the movements of respiration, as we have seen in speaking of Fabricius, served a double, or rather a triple, purpose. In the first place the air introduced by breathing served to regulate, to maintain, and at the same time to temper, to refrigerate the innate heat of the heart, that fire which, placed in the heart at the beginning, continued there all life long and was the one source of the warmth of the body. In the second place the pumping action of the chest served to introduce into the blood the air which was necessary for the generation in the left side of the heart of the vital spirits, which were thence distributed over the body by the arteries. In the third place the same action served to get rid of the fuliginous vapours, the products of the innate fire burning in the heart. Both the pure air engendering the vital spirits, and the foul vapours the effect of the heart's labours, were supposed to pass by the vein-like artery, the pulmonary vein, the one one way, the other the other.

The absurdity of supposing that the same channel could serve for these two currents is put forward by Harvey in his book as the first difficulty which meets one in considering the validity of the Galenic doctrines; but it was a difficulty which Fabricius did not feel or which at least lay lightly upon him.

With Harvey's demonstration all this view fell crumbling to the ground. It was seen that as the blood-stream swept through the lungs from the right to the left side of the heart a great change in the blood took place; from being venous it became arterial. But what the change exactly was, or how it took place, and what the connection was between the change in the blood and the movements of the lungs, and indeed what was the exact purpose of the bellows-like heaving and falling of the chest remained unsolved problems.

Van Helmont, as we have seen, if we may distinguish between his fourth and his fifth fermentation, thought that the blood in passing through the lungs suffered a fermentation by which it became lighter in colour and more volatile, a fermentation different from and introductory to that by which the vital spirits were engendered in the left ventricle, and across the septum in the right ventricle also. But he is not clear on this point, and in any case he seems to have attributed nothing to any mingling of the blood in the veins with the air in the lungs.

When we come to Borelli we pass at once into a clear understanding of the problem so far as the mechanical side of it is concerned. He applied to the mechanics of breathing the new knowledge which had been arrived at on the one hand of muscular contraction, and on the other hand of the pressure and elasticity of the atmosphere, and so at once reached the truth that inspiration consists in the entrance of air by virtue of the pressure of the atmosphere into the chest enlarged by the muscular contraction of its walls, and expiration in the exit of the air so entering, mainly at least by cessation of contraction. Fabricius had, as we have seen, some sound views on this matter, but Borelli went far beyond him.

When he came to deal with the chemical aspects of breathing Borelli rejected instantly and peremptorily the old view that the movements of breathing were for the cooling and ventilation of the innate fire of the heart, or for expelling the vapours generated by such a fire.

In discussing the subject in his book he lays down by the help of formulae and figures certain propositions concerning the laws of mixture of the minute particles of diverse fluids exposed in certain channels to certain pressures; and he finishes his exposition with the following words:

"I have expounded the above matters because eminent "anatomists have thought that breathing was instituted in "order that the chief parts of the blood (namely the serous "and coloured parts as well as the chylous material together "with the lymph) may be completely mixed in the lungs so "that for instance the minutest particles of the one may come "in contact with and receive among themselves the minutest "particles of the rest. And they think that this is effected by "the repeated rythmic pressure exerted by the inflated vessels.

"Therefore after my wont, without mentioning any names, I "will, in the interests of truth, expound the reasons which "render such an opinion doubtful." And this he goes on to do.

Now Malpighi, in the letter to Borelli in which he announced his discovery of the true structure of the lung, and which Borelli at the time loaded with praise, had ventured to put forward just such an explanation as that given above of the use of the lungs. It is his old friend Malpighi whom Borelli is here attacking.

And Malpighi, in his autobiography finished just before his death, and published by the Royal Society in 1697 as part of his posthumous works, in describing how his little tracts were received by the learned world, refers to the matter in the following way:

"You will wonder, Reader, when I tell you that the most "learned Giovanni Alphonso Borelli, whom I a little while back "spoke of as most anxious that my Letters should be pub-"lished, now breaks out into opposition to and severe criticism "of my views. The reason which has led him to do this is "because the literary intercourse which existed between us "having been broken off he became so inflamed with anger "against me and mine that in the book which he composed "in his last declining years, namely the one on the movement "of animals, he seized the opportunity of disproving my "opinions. In this book, he, without mentioning my name, "attacks with many arguments the use assigned by me to "the lungs." He then in turn refutes Borelli's arguments; apparently he remained by his old opinion until his death.

Borelli sums up his exposition of the erroneous views put forward concerning the purpose of breathing as follows:

"It is clear from what has been said that the use of "breathing is not the cooling of the excessive heat of the "heart, nor the ventilation of the vital flame, nor the mixture "of the heterogeneous parts of the blood brought about by "the pressure of the inflated vesicles of the lungs, nor merely "the passage of blood from the right to the left ventricle of "the heart in order that the circulation may be carried on. "But so great a machinery of vessels and organs of the lungs "must have been instituted for some grand purpose; and that

"we will try to expound, if possible, though we shall stammer
"as we go along."

He remarks that, in spite of the experiment that air blown
through a tube into the bronchial tubes does not enter the
pulmonary vein, many authors maintain, and justly maintain,
that air does somehow find its way from the lungs into the
blood. These authors suppose for this purpose the existence
of minute pores leading from the interior of the lungs into the
blood vessels. Such a supposition, however, is, in his opinion,
not necessary, since air dissolved in liquids can pass through
membranes, and there is always in the bronchial passages
some fluid in which the air might be dissolved.

He goes on to insist that "air taken in by breathing is the
"chief cause of the life of animals," far more essential than
the working of the heart and the circulation of the blood.
A frog will live after its heart has been wholly cut away, and
insects may be divided into pieces and yet live for a while.
The stoppage of breathing, on the other hand, brings about
in all cases the cessation of life.

"The experiment which proves most completely the truth
"of the assertion (that air is necessary to life) is the sudden
"removal of air by Boyle's pneumatic machine, or better still
"by the Torricellian vacuum with the help of mercury.
"Animals of all kinds shut up in such a vacuum immediately
"fall down dead; but if the air be instantly renewed with
"care, may be brought to life again."

He recognized that particles of the air taken into the lungs
enter in and become mixed with the blood. But true to his
position as a physicist dealing only with problems capable of
being solved with mathematical certitude, and refusing to
attempt to solve problems in any other way, he rejects all
vague chemical suggestions as to particular chemical substances being drawn from the air and mixed with the blood.
"The particles of the air mixed with the blood do not increase
"its flexibility, nor do they produce an effervescence in the
"heart by reason of their elastic force or of their nitrous
"nature." He invents a physical hypothesis of molecular
movement. He supposes that the entrance of air into the
blood produces continual delicate oscillations (*continuae*

motionis tremulae), which like the pendulum of a clock regulate all animal actions.

This exposition by Borelli appeared in print when his book was published in 1680–1; but, as we have already said, much which is to be found in the book had been publicly taught by him many years before, while he was at Pisa. Since, as he himself admits, he rarely quoted authorities, it is difficult in many cases to decide whether the view which Borelli is expounding is really his own, reached by him at an early date, or has been taken from some other author who had put it forth before Borelli's book was finished for the press. And, as we have seen, he never really finished the book; he continued labouring to improve it until almost the day of his death. We may however conclude from the quotations just given that he was acquainted with the views put forward during his lifetime by the English School of which I am about to speak; and we may also conclude that he rejected those views. To these we must now turn.

Robert Boyle, as all know, busied himself with the new views as to the weight and pressure of air introduced by the observations of Galileo, Torricelli, and Pascal, by which the old plenum doctrine of Descartes was overthrown. With his new pneumatical engine, or air-pump (which von Guericke had just before introduced), he made many researches on the spring or *elater* of air.

He shewed in 1660 that even in a partial vacuum brought about by his air-pump, and much sooner in a more complete one, flame was extinguished and life soon came to an end; the candle went out and the mouse or the sparrow died.

This experiment, which is referred to in the quotation from Borelli given above, must be regarded as the fundamental experiment in the physiology of respiration. It shewed not only that the thing called air, and not merely the movement of the chest in breathing, was essential to the due effect of breathing, but also that the change whatever it might be which was effected by breathing was identical with that which was going on in the burning of a candle.

The next step was taken by Robert Hooke. This man, of singular ingenuity, born in 1635 and dying in 1702, held for many years, from 1664 until his death, the office of curator of experiments to the newly founded Royal Society, having been some time previously assistant to Boyle. He was one of the earliest and most zealous users of the newly invented microscope, and in his *Micrographia*, published by the Royal Society in 1667, records his numerous 'Observations made on Minute Bodies of very varied kinds by Magnifying Glasses.'

As Curator to the Royal Society it was his duty to perform experiments before the Fellows at their meetings, and these experiments, such was the versatile ability of the Curator, were very diverse in kind—physical, chemical, and physiological.

At their meeting of Oct. 24, 1667, he delighted the Fellows of the Society with an experiment on artificial respiration, an account of which is given in No. 28 of the *Philosophical Transactions*. The experiment of artificial respiration had often been done before. Vesalius tells us how he used to perform it, and points out how the beat of the heart and arteries grew faint and almost ceased when the action of the bellows was stopped, and how it revived again with great vigour so soon as inflation was begun again. But no one had drawn from the experiment the important conclusion which Hooke drew.

In the first place having widely opened the thorax of a dog, he shewed that the animal could be kept alive by artificial respiration in absence of all movements of the chest wall. This proved, and the point had been previously doubtful, or at least not unreservedly accepted, that the whole of the essential business of respiration is carried on in the lungs, that the movements of the chest are useful only so far as they bring about the changes, the alternate expansion and collapse of the lungs.

In the second place, and this was really the important part of the experiment, he shewed that the animal could almost equally well be kept alive without any movement of the lung. He kept the lung motionless but thoroughly distended by maintaining a powerful blast with the bellows, the air driven in escaping continually through minute holes pricked in the lung. This shewed that the mere movement of the lungs in breathing which had of old been thought to be the essential factor in respiration was an incidental and not a necessary feature of the business. The essential feature was a supply of fresh air adequate to keep up the resulting change in the blood. The qualities, whatever they might be, by assuming which blood passing through the lungs became arterial and thus fit to nourish the body were imparted to the blood not by movement but by the mere exposure of the blood to air, that is to fresh air. The concussions, which it had been supposed by some were given to the column of blood by the movements of breathing, had nothing to do with the matter, nor indeed had movement any real share in the business. The secret of the change lay in the mere exposure of the blood to fresh air, to air made fresh, in natural breathing, by the bellows-like action of the chest. And Hooke at the close of the experiment asked the pertinent question "whether suffer-"ing the (venous) blood to circulate through a vessel so "that it may be openly exposed to the fresh air may not "suffice (instead of lungs and breathing) for the life of the "animal?"

The next step was taken by Richard Lower. I have already referred to this singularly able man, the henchman of the fashionable Willis, whose false fame in large measure rested on Lower's careful, unacknowledged work.

Born in Cornwall in 1631, educated at Westminster School in London and afterwards at Oxford, he stayed in the latter city for some years, while Willis was Professor.

In 1665 he created quite an excitement by his experiments on transfusion; through these he became for a while the talk of the town. The inordinate hopes which were raised by this new method were never realized; but the fact that such experiments were at that time made is a striking proof of what a revolution had been effected in men's views as to the circulation of the blood in the thirty-seven years which had passed since Harvey's book was published. Before the doctrine of the circulation of the blood had been established, to prolong life or cure disease by injecting blood into a blood vessel would have seemed the height of absurdity.

The fame of his transfusion seems to have brought Lower from Oxford to practise in London, where especially after Willis's death in 1675 he became very popular; but his pronounced political attitude, he was a fervent whig, stood in his way, his practice 'fell off' and he died in anything but prosperous circumstances in 1690.

In 1669 he published his *Tractatus de corde*. In this he not only gave a much more accurate description than anyone had given before of the structure of the heart, including the distribution of its nerves, but he also gave an account of the physiology of the heart, in which he completed and extended Harvey's exposition with the help of all the new exact physics which had come to hand since Harvey wrote his work. He gave more accurate measurements than Harvey had published (Harvey as we know had made many observations in addition to those recorded in his book, observations which he promised to publish but never did) concerning the amount of work done by the heart, and the velocity of the flow in the arteries. He recognized the meaning of the stout walls of the arteries and the thin coats of the veins. He noticed that when one carotid was ligatured the other beat more forcibly on account of the greater amount of blood thrown into it. He produced ascites by ligaturing the vena cava high up, and intravascular clotting by injecting milk. He was aware that the heart would beat for a while cut away from all its connections. In short he obtained at that early date a rough, perhaps, but true view of most of the main facts of the circulation. As a Fellow of the Royal Society he was of the opinion that new truths were to be reached mainly by way of experiment, and as a physiologist he like Harvey sought for truth in experiments on living animals. And his experiments led him to truth. His exposition of the circulation though less formal than that of his contemporary Borelli, for Borelli was teaching while Lower was experimenting and practising, not bristling as does Borelli's with mathematical formulae and scholastic theorems and lemmas, comes in many respects much nearer the truth, is much more like a modern exposition, and may with profit be read at the present day.

But it is not to Lower's views on the heart and circulation

that I wish now to call attention. In his work on the heart there is included the account of experiments having results fundamental in the history of respiration.

It was known of course of old that venous blood was dark and arterial bright, but the change was thought to take place in the heart, on the left side of the heart; and this view was maintained even after the circulation through the lungs had been accepted (though van Helmont seems to have caught sight of the truth that the change might take place in the lungs). Moreover the change in colour was thought to be only a superficial accompaniment of profound differences between the blood in the arteries and the blood in the veins.

Lower's careful quantitative determinations and calculations of the flow of blood through the heart raised as he says doubts in his mind as to "whether there could be that great "difference between venous and arterial blood which the "vulgar think."

He suspected that the change of colour took place in the lungs as the contents of the pulmonary artery found their way into the pulmonary veins, and that it was due simply to the exposure of the blood to the air in the lungs. But so long as he made observations on natural breathing he failed to satisfy himself of the correctness of his supposition.

Hooke's experiment on artificial respiration gave him the opportunity he desired. Examining the lungs of an animal kept alive by artificial respiration after the chest had been opened, he had no difficulty in ascertaining that the blood in the pulmonary veins long before it reached the heart was florid in colour. He further saw that when the artificial respiration was stopped, when no fresh air was driven into the lungs, when the animal was suffocated, the blood in the pulmonary veins and in the left side of the heart became dark and venous. He took dark venous blood from the vena cava, and injected it artificially through the lungs. He found that so long as insufflation of the lungs was kept up the blood ran out by the pulmonary veins florid in colour, but ran out dark and unchanged if no fresh air was driven in to the lungs.

He concluded that the change in colour was due simply to the blood being exposed in the lungs to air; and he was confirmed in this conclusion by observing the fact that a clot of dark venous blood soon becomes florid on the upper surface where it is exposed to the air; and that if the cake be turned upside down the under dark surface also soon becomes florid.

And he at once took the next step and drew the further conclusion that the change in colour was due not to mere exposure alone but to the blood taking up some of the air. Arterial blood, according to him, differs from venous in that it contains air; as the florid arterial blood passes from the body air escapes from it and it becomes dark and venous; as the dark venous blood passes through the pulmonary circulation it takes up air again and once more becomes florid and arterial.

It is this continual entrance of fresh air into the blood which renders fresh air so necessary for the maintenance of life. "Were it not for this we should breathe as well in the "most filthy prison as among the most delightful pastures." The same fresh air is as much needed for our breathing as for the burning of a flame, "in fact where a fire burns readily, "there can we easily breathe."

Lower speaks only of air being taken up as air, and as we have seen Borelli had also come to the conclusion that air is taken up by the blood in the lungs; but he, writing towards the end of the seventies, might have been acquainted with Lower's results. Neither one nor the other alludes to the possibility of a part of the air only being taken. It was the common opinion of the time and one which lasted for long afterwards that air, the air of the atmosphere, was a single substance not a mixture of two or more things, though it was admitted that in the atmosphere there existed besides the air proper, or pure air, suspended as it were in this, a number of particles of a different and probably varied nature.

Both Lower and Borelli seem to have thought that it was the air proper, and not any special particles in it, which passing into the blood brought about the change of colour. Hooke, in his *Micrographia* in 1667, treating of charcoal and speculating concerning flame, propounds the view that it is due to action of a part of the air which he calls a 'menstruum,' "a substance inherent in and mixt with the air, that is like,

"if not the very same with that which is fixt in Salt-peter."
But he does not go beyond this, and does not apply the same
view to breathing.

It was left for a countryman of Lower, for one belonging as
he did to the University of Oxford, to take the next step in
the physiology of respiration and to bring forward reasons
for thinking that in breathing only a part of the air, not
the whole air, not the air proper, was taken up into the
blood.

John Mayow, coming like Lower of a Cornish family, was
born in London in 1643, the year before van Helmont died.
Admitted a scholar at Wadham College, Oxford, he became
in due time a Fellow of All Souls. Devoted as he was to
science, physic was not his profession; he took a degree in
law "and became noted for his practice therein, especially in
"the summer time at Bath." Yet to judge from his works
one would have thought that the whole of his time at Oxford
had been given up to continued research. In 1668, just four
years before Sylvius's death, he published, while as yet a
young man of twenty-five years, a little work containing four
tracts, (1) *De sal nitro et spiritu nitro aereo*, (2) *De respiratione*,
(3) *De respiratione fœtus in utero et ovo*, (4) *De motu musculari
et spiritibus animalibus*. He eventually migrated to London
and in 1678 was admitted a Fellow of the Royal Society. In
the following year he died in Covent Garden at the all too
early age of thirty-five, "having been married a little before
"not altogether to his content."

Mayow's contribution to our knowledge of respiration was
this. He shewed that it was not the whole air which was
necessary for respiration, and which was used for respiration,
but a particular part only of the air; and, as we shall see, by
this particular part, though he called it by a different name,
he meant what we now call oxygen.

The formation of nitre in heaps of decomposing animal and
vegetable matter, and the properties of nitre or saltpetre,
especially as the constituent of gunpowder, had for a long
time excited the interests of chemists. Nitre was made the
pivot of various chemical theories and ideas. "Nitre, which
"has made as much noise in philosophy as in war."

Sylvius in treating of respiration, of the mechanics of which he gives a fair description, and concerning which he had reached the conclusion that in breathing air passes from the lungs into the blood and produces a notable change in it, has the following remark. "By what power however, or in "what manner or way the inspired air so alters the blood, is "not equally clear. I think it is brought about by reason of "there being dispersed in the air nitrous and sub-acid parts "able to condense the effervescing and rarefied blood and to "gently restrain its ebullition. I distinguish however between "the sub-acid and the nitrous parts of the air, since the sub-"acid parts are for the most part simple, but the nitrous on "the contrary are compound, composed of acids if you like, "though not with any you please, but also of oily parts and "lixivious salts, as is clearly proved by the artificial (*i.e.* "chemical) synthesis and analysis of nitre."

Whether Sylvius wrote the above as the result of his own researches or whether he had heard of Mayow's inquiries is not certain; but in any case Sylvius's obscure views are very different from what we shall see to be the definite and clear conceptions of Mayow.

In the introduction to his tract on sal-nitrum Mayow undertakes to prove,

"That this air which surrounds us, and which, since by its "tenuity it escapes the sharpness of our eyes, seems to those "who think about it to be an empty space, is impregnated "with a certain universal salt, of a nitro-saline nature, that "is to say with a vital, fiery and in the highest degree fer-"mentative spirit."

It is this which he calls sal-nitro-aereum or spiritus nitro-aereus, or sometimes igneo-aereus.

Mayow was a chemist, far more of a chemist that Lower or Hooke, perhaps even more distinctly a chemist than Boyle; he had doubtless read carefully the works of Sylvius and van Helmont, and had probably repeated many of their experiments. He uses the current terms of the chemists of the period; and in reference to this it may be well to note that the word 'salt' had not yet acquired the limited meaning afterwards attached to it; it was still often used to denote any substance (whether elementary, as we should now say, or compound) not distinctly metallic, or distinctly liquid.

Mayow first expounds the nature of nitre. The common method at that time of preparing nitre was to allow heaps of vegetable matter to decompose with exposure to the air, and then to dissolve out and crystallize the potash nitre so formed. He says that it is derived partly from the air and partly from the earth. There is the *sal fixum* or sal alkali or, as we now say, potash; this distinctly comes from the earth. Besides this there is the *spiritus acidus* or, as we now say, nitric acid.

For a while he thought that the whole of this spiritus acidus was derived from the air, that it existed distributed throughout the atmosphere divided into extremely minute particles. But this seemed incompatible with the well-known fact that the spiritus acidus is a corrosive liquid, extinguishing flame and destructive to life. He concludes therefore that part only of the acid exists in the atmosphere, and that part is his sal-nitro-aereum or spiritus nitro-aereus.

In attempting to lay hold of the nature of this nitro-aereal agent he first reminds his readers that a certain part of the air is necessary for the maintenance of combustion. He says:

"In the first place it must, I take it, be granted that "something in the air, whatever it be, is necessary for the "burning of every flame. This Boyle's experiments have "placed beyond doubt. For these shew that a lighted candle "goes out much more quickly in a glass flask empty of air "than in the same vessel full of air, a clear proof that the "flame, enclosed in the flask, goes out not because it is "suffocated by its own smoke, as some have thought, but "because it is deprived of its aereal sustenance or food "(*pabulum*). For since there is more room for the reception "of the smoke in the flask when it is exhausted of air than "when it is full of air, the candle ought to go out more "quickly in the latter than in the former, if its going out was "merely due to the smoke.

"Moreover sulphureous (*i.e.* combustible, he uses the time-"honoured Valentinian nomenclature of the different natures "of things) matter, of whatever kind, when placed in a flask "exhausted of air, cannot be ignited either by burning charcoal

"or red-hot iron, or by the sun's rays concentrated by means
"of a burning-glass. So that there cannot be now the slight-
"est doubt but that certain aereal particles are altogether
"necessary for the lighting of fire; and indeed our opinion is
"that these same particles play the chief part in igniting fire,
"and that the form of flame depends mainly on these particles
"being agitated in a most destructive manner, as I shall shew
"more fully later on.

"But it must not be thought that the igneo-aereal food (of
"flame) is air itself; it is only a more active and subtle part
"of it. For a candle enclosed in a flask goes out although
"there is still contained in the flask an amply abundance of
"air. Now we cannot suppose that the particles of air which
"existed in the flask were destroyed by the burning of the
"candle or that they escaped and got away, for such par-
"ticles are unable to pass through the glass. Moreover it
"is not probable that those igneo-aereal particles are a sort
"of perfected nitre, as the common opinion runs, for as
"has been shewn above it is not the very whole of the
"nitre but only a certain part of it which is derived from
"the air."

He then goes on to shew that the particles of air, forming
the more active and subtlé part of air which is thus necessary
for combustion, exist in nitre and indeed constitute its "more
"active and fiery part." For sulphur when mixed with nitre
will burn in the absence of air, in a vacuum for instance, or
under water. "Thus a squib made of gunpowder of which
"nitre is an important constituent will burn right away
"under water."

For every combustion there is needed on the one hand
sulphureous (combustible) material, and on the other hand
igneo-aereal particles. Now there are no sulphureous particles in nitre, hence nitre will not burn by itself. But nitre
as just stated when mixed with sulphureous particles burns
most readily, even without the access of air.

He concludes that the aereal part of nitre is nothing else
than the igneo-aereal particles of which he has been speaking
as essential to combustion; these particles exist, not in the sal
alkali part of the nitre, but in the spiritus acidus part; and he

enters into an explanation why the whole nitre, spiritus acidus and sal alkali together, is better suited for burning than the spiritus acidus itself, though this really contains the elements essential to combustion.

It is obvious from the above that Mayow by his nitro-aereal or igneo-aereal salt or spirit meant nothing less than that which we for a hundred years or more have been calling *oxygen*. And he thus, with clear insight, sums up the conditions necessary for combustion to take place:

"Concerning fire (combustion) it must be noted that for the "ignition of this it is necessary that igneo-aereal particles "should either pre-exist in the thing to be burnt or should be "supplied from the air. Gunpowder is very easily burnt by "itself by reason of the igneo-aereal particles existing in it. "Vegetables are burnt partly by means of the igneo-aereal "particles existing in them, partly by help of those brought "to them from the air. Purified sulphureous matter, on the "contrary, can be burnt only with the help of igneo-aereal "particles brought to it by the air."

He also recognized that in combustion the igneo-aereal particles enter into combination with the substance burnt. In the course of this discussion on burning he makes the following very remarkable reflection. He was writing in 1668. Many years afterwards in 1697 Stahl, as I have said, introduced the phlogiston theory. The essence of that theory was the view that when a combustible body, a phlogisticated body, underwent combustion, phlogiston departed from it; the body suffered a loss, it became dephlogisticated. The world had to wait for nearly a hundred years after Stahl until Lavoisier overthrew the theory by proving that in combustion a body suffered not loss but gain: the metal burnt into a metallic oxide increased in weight. That is what Mayow said more than a hundred years before Lavoisier, many years before Stahl:

"Nor must the following point be passed over, that anti-"monium burned by the sun's rays (collected by a burning-"glass) increases considerably in weight; as may be proved "by experiment (*i.e.* by actual weighing). Now we can hardly "conceive that the increase of weight of the antimonium

"arises from anything else than from the igneo-aereal par-
"ticles inserted into it during the calcination."

What a zigzag path, how unlike a straight line, is man's
progress in search of truth. Here is Mayow reaching a point
far ahead, and Boyle a little later had grasped the same fact;
Stahl drags, or seems to drag, the whole world of thought
back; and more than a hundred years afterwards Lavoisier
reaches the same point as Mayow. How true it is that the
value of a truth is not absolute; there is a time and a place
for everything, including a new truth. If a discovery is made
before its time, it withers up barren, without progeny, as did
Mayow's.

Having thus developed his views as to the nature of combustion Mayow went on to identify burning and breathing.
Both, he said, consist in the consumption of the igneo-aereal
particles of the air:

"If a small animal and a lighted candle be shut up in the
"same vessel, the entrance into which of air from without be
"prevented, you will see in a short time the candle go out;
"nor will the animal long survive its funeral torch. Indeed
"I have found by observation that an animal shut up in a
"flask together with a candle will continue to breathe for
"not much more than half the time than it otherwise would,
"that is, without the candle.

"Nor is it to be supposed that the animal in such a case is
"suffocated by the smoke of the candle, since if the flame be
"supplied by the burning of spirits of wine no smoke is
"produced (and yet the animal dies); moreover when a candle
"is used the animal lives for some time after the candle has
"gone out and its smoke has disappeared, so that we cannot
"suppose that it is suffocated by the smoke.

"The reason why the animal can live some time after the
"candle has gone out seems to be as follows. The flame of the
"candle needs for its maintenance a continuous and at the
"same time a sufficiently full and rapid stream of nitro-aereal
"particles. Whence it comes about that if the succession of
"nitro-aereal particles be interrupted, even for a moment, or
"if these are not supplied in adequate quantity, the flame
"presently sinks and goes out. Hence, so soon as the igneo-

"aereal particles begin to reach the flame scantily and slowly,
"it is soon extinguished. For animals, on the other hand, a
"lesser store of the aereal food is sufficient, and one supplied
"at intervals, so that the animal can be sustained by the
"aereal particles remaining after the candle has gone out.
"Here it may be remarked that the movements (expansions)
"of the collapsed lungs not a little help towards the sucking
"in of aereal particles which may remain in the said flask,
"and towards transferring them into the blood of the breath-
"ing animal. Whence it comes about that the animal does not
"perish until just before the aereal particles are wholly ex-
"hausted. And hence it is that air in which an animal is
"suffocated is diminished in volume more than twice as
"much as that in which a candle goes out."

This latter sentence refers to another aspect of the matter.
Physicists were then much exercised and Boyle's experiments
in particular had led to much discussion about the 'spring'
(*elater*) of air—the elastic force (*vis elastica*) of air, and the
pressure of air.

Mayow observes that when a candle is burnt in a closed
vessel over water, the water rises after the primary depression,
due to expansion from heating, has passed off; the burning
has deprived the air of some of its elastic force. He finds
by experiment that exactly the same thing takes place in
breathing. When a small animal is made to breathe in a
closed vessel standing over water the water rises. When a
mouse is put inside a cupping-glass, placed over a piece
of wet bladder stretched out loosely, over the wide mouth of
a bottle for instance, the bladder bulges up into the cupping-
glass. "I have found," says he, "by experimenting with
"various animals that air (of a closed vessel in which the
"animal is allowed to remain until it dies for want of air)
"is by the breathing of animals reduced in volume by
"about $\frac{1}{14}$th."

By such experiments as these "it is manifest," says he,
"that air is deprived of its elastic force by the breathing of
"animals just in the same way that it is by the burning of
"a flame. We may infer that animals and fire deprive the
"air of particles of the same kind."

Mayow, as I have said and indeed as we have seen, was essentially a chemist, but he was also well versed in the new physical learning of the time. It was only natural that he should be fascinated with the elastic force which he believed to be possessed to a peculiar degree by his igneo-aereal particles. He attributed an exaggerated importance to this elastic force. He enters into a long disquisition about it, and offers by means of it an explanation of the explosive force of gunpowder. As we have already hinted and as we shall later on clearly see, the chemical meaning of Mayow's discoveries was soon forgotten. His chemical exposition was premature. But his physical exposition fell on congenial soil. His igneo-aereal particles continued to be spoken of after him, not with the chemical properties which he attributed to them, but with the physical properties only, simply as the elastic particles of air.

Mayow however was not merely a chemist or a physicist, he was above all things a physiologist. In his third tract, 'On Respiration,' he gives in the first place an exposition of the mechanics of breathing, an exposition clearer and better, more exact and more true than that of Borelli, free from Borelli's pedantic formalities, an exposition which might almost find its place in a text-book of the present day.

He explains that air enters the lungs during breathing simply and solely because the pressure of the atmosphere or the elastic force of the atmosphere drives air in to fill up the increased space afforded by the enlarged and dilated thorax. And he points out how the structure of the lung, as made clear by Malpighi (seven years before he was writing), is admirably fitted by its vesicles and tubes for such a purpose. He illustrates his meaning by the well-known experiment of a collapsed bladder expanding in a closed vessel as the air is exhausted; and makes a quaint model of the chest and lungs by means of a bladder inserted in the cavity of a pair of bellows so that the mouth of the bladder is continuous with the nozzle of the bellows. When the bellows are expanded air rushes into the bladder and fills it, when the bellows are brought down the air is driven out again from the bladder.

Asking the question how the chest is enlarged during inspiration, he answers by the raising of the ribs and the descent of the diaphragm; the ribs are raised by the intercostal muscles, both external and internal; here he takes a side in a controversy which nearly a century later became acute between Haller and Hamberger, and has from time to time risen up again ever since. The diaphragm descends by virtue of its own contraction. Expiration he argues is in ordinary breathing the mere passive result of relaxation, the ribs falling back into their place and the contents of the abdomen pushing up the diaphragm. And he enters into several minor details, such for instance as the nature of the articulation of the ribs to the spine, by which their movements are facilitated. The whole account, as I have just said, might almost have been written at the present day.

He then proceeds to the larger question, What is the use of breathing? What effect is produced by breathing?

He ridicules the old and as yet still common view that breathing serves for cooling the heart. The blood and its fermentations, he says, seem to need heat rather than cold. And violent exercise, even one so brief that the blood has not time to get overheated, is followed by a much more intense respiration than is the highest fever.

He rejects the opinion, which he affirms to be even more common, that breathing is to facilitate the passage of the blood from the right to the left side of the heart. It is absurd, he says, to suppose that such an elaborate mechanism is needed for a mere transit. And indeed that the movements of breathing are not necessary for the transit is shewn by the simple experience that "when you hold your breath as long "as you can the finger on the pulse will tell you that blood "is still rapidly passing into the arteries," and therefore must have made the transit through the quiescent lungs.

Still another opinion that the blood is agitated, comminuted and broken as it were into very minute particles, is also according to him wrong, for any air would produce this mere mechanical effect, and air vitiated by some contagion or air which had been breathed over and over again would be equally good for respiration.

"And indeed if the need of breathing only arose,· as some
"have thought, in order that the mass of the blood should
"be thoroughly shaken by the movements of the lungs and
"broken up as it were into extremely minute parts, there
"would be no reason why an animal should so quickly expire
"when shut up in a flask in the manner stated. For the air
"in the flask even after the death of the animal is quite as
"well fitted as before for the inflation of the lungs and so
"for the comminution of the blood. For since that air is still
"subject to the pressure of almost the whole atmosphere,
"there is nothing to prevent its being driven into the dilated
"thorax of the animal, it being this, as I have elsewhere said,
"on which the inflation of the lungs depends."

No, he says, it is evident that something belonging to the
air, whatever it be, something necessary for sustaining life
passes from the air into the blood. Hence air which has been
already breathed, and which has in consequence been exhausted of those vital particles, is no longer fit for being
breathed again.

"On the one hand it clearly appears that animals exhaust
"the air of certain vital particles which are of an elastic
"nature. On the other hand there cannot be the slightest
"doubt but that some constituent of the air absolutely
"necessary to life enters into the blood in the act of breathing.

"We have no right to deny the entrance of air into the
"blood because on account of the bluntness of our senses we
"cannot actually see the vessels by which it makes its
"entrance. For other ducts, which serve to carry denser
"liquids, are not visible to the eyes until their several hair-
"like passages, after running a certain distance, join together
"to form a notable canal. What eye has ever been sharp
"enough to see the first beginnings of the lymphatic, or of
"the lacteal vessels, or even of the veins?" He does not seem
to have read Malpighi's second tract, and Leeuenhoek had
not yet made his more convincing observations. "How much
"less are we likely to see these aereal ducts, which must be
"very short and exceedingly delicate. For these passages are
"not like the others, passages becoming joined together after
"running separately for some distance; they only have to

"traverse the membranes of the lungs, each following a very
"short and obscure path. For in order that the aereal par-
"ticles should mix with the mass of blood in a state of fine
"division and in a most intimate manner, it is necessary that
"they should enter the blood through channels or rather
"orifices almost infinite in number, distributed here and there
"over the whole mass of the lungs. And indeed in lungs which
"have been prepared and dissected, holes, almost without
"number, like most minute points may be seen with the aid
"of the microscope. Whether however those points are the
"mouths of capillary air tubes or of vessels opening into the
"blood cannot be determined for certain.

"Let us inquire in the next place what is that constituent
"of the air which thus passes into the blood, which is so
"necessary for sustaining life that we cannot live for even
"a moment of time without it. And indeed it is very probable
"that certain particles of a nitro-saline nature, and those very
"subtle, nimble, and of very great fermentative power, are
"separated from the air by the aid of the lungs and introduced
"into the mass of the blood. And so necessary for life of every
"kind is that aereal salt (constituent) that not even plants
"can grow in earth the access of air to which is shut off. But
"if that same earth be exposed to air and so forthwith im-
"pregnated with that fecundating salt, it at once becomes
"fit again for growing. It is clear that even the very plants
"seem to have some need of breathing, some need of drawing
"air into themselves.

"What part however this aereal salt plays in animal life
"it is not easy to understand. It is at all events probable
"that the nitro-aereal spirit, mixed with salino-sulphureous
"particles of the blood, excites in it a needed fermentation.
"We must not however suppose that the effervescence of the
"blood takes place in the heart alone; it takes place also in
"the pulmonary vessels before the blood reaches the heart,
"and afterwards in the arteries, no less than in the heart
"itself."

The word 'effervescence' shews that he had read Sylvius.
Possibly, or perhaps we may rather say probably, his acute
mind had, pondering much over fermentations, begun to

grasp some new ideas about these mysterious processes, and had he lived we might have learnt from him things which did not come until much later.

Touching thus upon fermentation, he turns aside to note that he is not forgetful of that 'fermentum' of a mysterious character supposed to exist in the left ventricle, the ferment of van Helmont's fifth digestion; but he scornfully rejects the idea. Then he passes on to have a tilt with Descartes, who, great philosopher, but amateur physiologist, as he was, had not as we have seen grasped the force of Harvey's arguments, and contended against Harvey that the beat of the heart was an expansion due to the rarefaction of the ventricular contents. Mayow had no difficulty in following Harvey and Lower in the proof that the blood was driven out of the heart by the contraction of the muscular walls. The heart, he says, is nothing but a muscle, very little different in its action from other muscles. And he clenches his argument against Descartes with two remarkable experiments. "If in the heart "of an animal just dead, filled not with blood, but with water "or some simple liquid, you excite a movement like that "which takes place in systole, the contents of the ventricle are "forthwith ejected, not indeed by reason of a fermentative "explosion, for such in this case certainly cannot take place, "but simply because the ventricles are contracted." Besides it is very certain that the movement of the heart can not be due to the rarefaction of the blood; for sometimes the heart, cut clean out of the body, may be seen to beat, although all the blood has already been driven out of the ventricles.

He then goes on to ask the question why death follows suppression of breathing.

"Life, unless I mistake, consists in the distribution of "animal spirits, for the supply of which the beating of the "heart and the flow of blood to the brain are absolutely "necessary. And breathing seems especially to assist the beat "of the heart, in a manner elsewhere described. Now it is "very probable that this aereal salt is wholly necessary for all "muscular movement, so that without it the beat of the heart "cannot take place. For we have reason to think that the "sudden contraction of a muscle is due to particles of two

"different kinds mixing with each other, and mutually acting
"upon each other. Now we cannot suppose that both kinds
"of particles, the effervescence of which gives rise to the
"contraction of muscles, can come from the mass of the blood,
"for liquids which are derived from the same source unite
"again without any effervescence. So that it seems that
"something extraneous is requisite for bringing about the
"ebullition which leads to muscular movement.

"We may therefore suppose that the nitro-saline particles
"derived from the inspired air supply the one class of motive
"particles which, meeting with the other, salino-sulphureous
"particles furnished by the mass of the blood, but dwelling
"in the motor structures, excite that effervescence which
"gives rise to the muscular contraction, as we have fully
"shewn elsewhere.

"The movement of the heart is carried out in the same way
"as in other muscles.

"Hence, when breathing is stopped, since that aereal salt,
"needful for all movement, is lacking, the beat of the heart
"and therefore the flow of blood to the brain are interrupted,
"and death necessarily follows."

This view of the use of the nitro-aereal particles naturally
leads to the corollary that "breathing is increased during
"violent exercise, not in order that a greater flow of blood
"may take place freely through the lungs, but in order to
"provide for the greater expenditure of the nitro-aereal salts
"in the many effervescences taking place in the contractions
"of the muscles."

His nitro-aereal hypothesis also enabled him to lay hold
of a sound theory of animal heat.

The union of the nitro-aereal particles (taken in by breathing) with the salino-sulphureous particles of the blood gives
rise to the heat of the blood. The greater heat which accompanies violent exercise is due to the greater supply of nitro-
aereal particles caused by the increased respiration. This
brings about an increased effervescence, and so an increase
of heat in the blood itself, but at the same time the heat is
also increased by the greater effervescence in the muscles
themselves.

It will thus be seen that Mayow had laid firmly hold of one factor of respiration, the entrance of something from the air of the pulmonary vesicles into the blood. He had not grasped the other factor now known to us, the exit of something from the blood into the pulmonary vesicles. He was only on the track of this. He says, "about expiration is to be noted that "this serves a further purpose, namely, that together with "the air driven out of the lungs, the vapour of the blood "agitated by the fermentation is blown away also." And he develops a theory, foreshadowing modern views, that it is a feature of the fermentative action of the nitro-aereal particles that the blood, when it comes back to the lungs as venous blood, having been deprived in the tissues of its nitro-aereal particles, is greedy of fresh particles of that kind, and so assists in drawing them into the blood out of the air of the lungs. So the fermentation of the blood is kept up by an automatic, self-regulating process.

I have ventured to dwell at such length on the writings of John Mayow because they afford a striking example of how the seed of truth fails to spring up into a plant unless it fall on congenial ground. By his nitro-aereal, or igneo-aereal particles, Mayow evidently meant what we now call oxygen. He saw that this formed only a part of the atmosphere, that it was essential for burning, that it was essential for all the chemical changes on which life depends, that it was absorbed into the blood from the lungs, carried by the blood to the tissues, and in the tissues was the pivot, the essential factor of the chemical changes by which the vital activities of this or that tissue are manifested. It was essential in muscle to the occurrence of muscular contractions, it was essential in the brain to the development of animal spirits.

This great truth was reached at a time when the men of chemistry were struggling with the spiritualistic fermentations of van Helmont on the one hand, and with the material effervescences of Sylvius on the other. It was reached by a young man of twenty-five years, who died a few years afterwards.

When we look at the portrait affixed to his book we see a face delicate in outline, yet with a firm mouth, the visage of a man who had spent his as yet short days in the quiet but earnest and unresting pursuit of truth amid the calm of academic retirement. His premature death bids us think that not long after he had made known the results of the labour of his early years, the beginnings of disease had already made his spirits droop and his hand hang heavy by his side. Otherwise he must have had something to say during the ten years which ran between the publication of his book and his death. Yet he was silent. Had his body been as strong as his mind was acute, had he lived to that ripe old age which was reached by many another leader in science, how different had been the story of chemical physiology.

But it was not to be. This bright school of English physiologists of the mid-seventeenth century—Boyle, Hooke, Lower, and Mayow, worthy children of the great Harvey—passed away, and for a long time none took their place. Though the physical and experimental work of the three former remained effective on men's minds, the chemical work of Mayow soon passed out of ken; a few passing references, and those for the most part feathered with scorn, to the supposed part played by nitrous particles in breathing, supply all that can be found in succeeding writers. The world had to wait for more than a hundred years till Mayow's thought arose again as it were from the grave in a new dress, and with a new name; and that which in the first years of the latter half of the seventeenth century as igneo-aereal particles shone out in a flash and then died away again into darkness, in the last years of the eighteenth century, as oxygen, lit a light which has burned, and which has lighted the world with increasing steadiness up to the present day.

LECTURE VIII

THE PHYSIOLOGY OF DIGESTION IN THE
EIGHTEENTH CENTURY

THE story, even in outline, of the progress of Physiology in the seventeenth century has in the preceding lectures been told in part only. Men's minds in that century were busy with problems of the animal body besides those of digestion and breathing; and I have yet to speak of other labours carried out by men on whom I have already dwelt, as well as of labours carried out by men of whom as yet I have said little or nothing. The division, however, of the labour of inquiry which the progress of science brought about as the years ran on renders it desirable that I should complete the stories of the progress of our knowledge of digestion and respiration, so far as I propose to carry them, before I speak of the advances made in other branches of physiology. I therefore propose to devote the present lecture to an account of the more striking researches in digestion which were carried out in the eighteenth century.

In a preceding lecture I spoke of two men as exerting, through their large chemical knowledge, an important influence on the ideas concerning the chemical problems of physiology at the latter end of the seventeenth and in the early years of the eighteenth century. On one of these, George Ernest Stahl, I have already dwelt.

The other man was Hermann Boerhaave, who was born on the 31st December 1668, four years before Sylvius's death, at Voorhout, near Leyden. The son of a minister he was brought up to follow his father's career, and his early years at the University of Leyden were largely given up to classical and oriental studies, though he at the same time eagerly took up mathematical physical learning in spite of this not being at that period in much favour at the University. In 1690 he became Doctor of Philosophy, choosing for the subject of his thesis 'The distinction between body and mind.' An illness, an obstinate ulcer of the thigh from which he suffered as a lad, seems to have turned his attention to medicine; and after his graduation while preparing himself by theological studies for his ordination and supporting himself (for his father died early) by teaching mathematics and by occasional literary work, he found time to study medicine and the ancillary sciences of chemistry and botany. Though he seems in these matters to have for the most part taught himself, attending but few lectures, he made such progress that in 1693 he obtained the degree of Doctor of Medicine, not however at Leyden but at the University of Harderwick. He intended at first to use this degree merely as an adjunct to his proper career as a clergyman; but having been led by his zeal for mathematics to refute, in a public conveyance, someone who was ignorantly declaiming against the doctrines of Spinoza, he acquired the reputation of being an adherent of that heterodox philosopher; and either because he feared that this taint of heresy might lead to difficulties about his ordination, or because the love of medical science was becoming stronger in him than the love of theology, he gave up the idea of the ministry and definitely threw himself into the practice of medicine. Thus, in the tangle of human events, Spinoza, by a roundabout way, gave Boerhaave, and through Boerhaave gave Haller, to medicine and to science.

His talents soon impressed the authorities of Leyden, and in 1701 he was placed in the Chair of Medicine left vacant by the death of Drelincourt in 1697. He was at first not made full professor, only lecturer. The power, however, which he shewed as a teacher rapidly made itself felt; students flocked to his lectures; and the authorities of the University, lest he should be tempted by offers from elsewhere, increased his emoluments, and gave scope to his unwearied energy and wide knowledge by placing him in more chairs than one. In 1709 he was made Ordinary Professor of Medicine and of Botany; in 1715 he became also Professor of Practical Medicine, and in 1716 Professor of Chemistry as well. Much sought after as a physician, acute at the bedside, brilliant as an expositor in the professorial chair, he was also a great teacher in the sense that in his daily intercourse with his pupils he was always ready to lay his mind open before them, and to let them share in his experience and in his thoughts. At Leyden he laboured all his life. He was more than once

Rector of the University; and although in 1729 he resigned the Chairs of Botany and Chemistry and allowed himself a leisure which he devoted chiefly to gardening in a country seat which he had bought, he still continued to teach medicine in spite of the diseases which were creeping upon him in his old age; and at Leyden he died in harness, full of honour and esteem, on the 23rd September 1738.

Boerhaave was in almost all respects a different man from Stahl. A learned scholar, and a sound scientific thinker, he was too all-round a man to be led away by any one idea however tempting; essentially eclectic in nature, he gathered truth from every source. Though living all his life in the University in which Sylvius had laboured so long and so strenuously, though himself versed above his fellows in chemical knowledge, his work on the subject being for years the great text-book of the subject, he did not exalt chemistry above anatomy or above physics. Though drawn to mathematics long before he thought of medicine, though an ardent student of Borelli's works and a pupil of the enthusiastic iatro-physicist Pitcairn, who in 1692 had been brought from Edinburgh to occupy for a brief period the Chair of Medicine at Leyden, he did not think that all the problems of the human body were such as could be solved by the mere use of formulae and the calculus. Though the intimate friend of the great anatomist Ruysch, he was not ready to admit with him that anatomical disposition supplied the answer to every physiological question. He made use of anatomy, of physics and of chemistry, but he never allowed one to exclude the other; he was ready to apply each one of these sciences to the elucidation of physiological phenomena; and the width and sagacity of his teaching are reflected in the work of his great pupil who followed after him, Albrecht von Haller, of whom I have soon to speak.

Boerhaave cannot be said to have made by his own researches any striking contribution to our knowledge of digestion. The part which he played was rather that of the sagacious eclectic teacher who has made himself well acquainted with all that others have done, and who criticizing, with wide knowledge, their various views, and pointing out where they are obviously wrong, gathers together what might seem to a sober mind the outcome of their various results.

Thus Boerhaave was not an extreme advocate either of the mechanical school or of the chemical fermentative school, but he admitted within limits the doctrines of each.

In his works, as for instance in his *Institutiones Medicae* (the first edition of which appeared in 1708), which remained for many years the common text-book of the schools, and the first part of which was a treatise on physiology, he recognizes that digestion is in part a solution of some of the constituents of the food by means of various juices. Saliva, the juice from the oesophagus, the gastric fluid, which consists in part of a viscous secretion poured out by the glands of the stomach, and in part of a thin fluid secreted by the arteries, the bile, the pancreatic juice, and the intestinal juice, each of these contributes to the result. But he regards the solution effected by means of these juices as of the nature of ordinary solution, not of a nature of fermentation. It is worth noticing that he denies the acidity of the gastric juice, and speaks of van Helmont's heresy on this point. Owing to the labours of Sylvius, Stahl, and others, men's ideas concerning acidity and alkalinity were becoming much more definite than they had been; coloured vegetable juices were coming into use as tests of one or the other; and Boerhaave, while denying the acidity of gastric juice, expresses his wonder that Sylvius, knowing as he did what an acid was, could ever have thought that pancreatic juice was acid. It may be added that Boerhaave regarding, in common with his contemporaries, the supply of nerves to the stomach as out of all proportion to the movements or sensations of that organ, believed that a nervous fluid having some share in the digestion of food was poured into the cavity of the stomach from the endings of the nerves.

This solution by means of juices was, however, in Boerhaave's opinion only a part of the digestive process. He joined with the mechanical school in believing that the more fluid and nutritious parts of various articles of food were expressed from them by trituration in the stomach. He expressly taught that the more solid and resisting framework of both animal and vegetable food was not digested at all; that digestion to a large extent consisted in this, that by the solvent action of the juices or by mechanical pressure the softer or more fluid material held by the framework was either dissolved or pressed out of it. In particular he thought that bones were not digested, only crushed, and pointed to the white excrement, the album.graecum, of dogs fed on bone as a proof of this.

Boerhaave's positive mode of thinking put him more or less in antagonism to the doctrines of fermentation, to which, as we have seen, the chemical school were so attached. He seems, moreover, to have distinguished between the chemical effervescence of Sylvius and true fermentation, such as that of wine. He regarded the action of the juices as a mere solution, not as a proper fermentation. Nevertheless he held that solution and trituration are, in digestion, aided by something else. He thought that in the stomach, which is a closed chamber, but with air present in it, the contents, exposed as they are to a considerable heat, do undergo "an incipient "fermentation, by means of which the chyle is impressed "with the primary principle of vitality."

Such were the doctrines taught by Boerhaave in the early years of the eighteenth century. They were very largely accepted, and indeed became the dominant views. We find almost the same teaching nearly fifty years afterwards when we come to Haller, of whom we must now speak.

The year 1757 may be regarded in a certain sense as a red letter year in the history of physiology, as marking an epoch, as indicating the dividing line between modern physiology and all that went before. It was the year in which the first volume of the *Elementa Physiologiae* of Haller was published, the eighth and last volume leaving the press in 1765.

Albrecht von Haller, descendant of an old Swiss family, was born at Bern on 18th October 1708. Precocious as a child he while yet young acquired a large knowledge both of literature and science, the former at first being dominant in him and leading him to the composition of many juvenile poems. Losing his father while yet a lad of thirteen, he continued his education for some time at Bern, but in 1723 entered the

University of Tübingen. In 1725, however, attracted by the renown of Boerhaave, he moved to Leyden; and there undoubtedly he laid the foundation of all his future work. At that time Boerhaave was in the fullness of his power, the ripeness of his experience adding more than might seem to be lost through the declining energy of advancing years; and he had now by his side the younger Albinus, Frederick Bernard Albinus, an accomplished and sagacious anatomist, who later on, in 1745, became Professor of Anatomy. Under these influences the younger Haller not only made rapid progress, but also had his versatile mind fixed in its proper direction. Taking in 1727 his degree as Doctor of Medicine at Leyden, upon a thesis in which he exposed the error of Coschwitz, professor at Halle, who had maintained that he had discovered a new duct of the submaxillary and sublingual glands, Haller spent some time in foreign travel. He visited Belgium, England, where he became the friend of Sir Hans Sloane, and France, and in 1728 took up for a while his abode at Basel, studying under the celebrated mathematician John Bernoulli, and beginning to devote his attention to systematic botany, at which he continued at intervals to labour all his life.

In 1730 he returned to his native city; and here for a while he taught anatomy and practised medicine, prosecuting all the while anatomical and physiological researches and spending his leisure hours partly in botanical explorations, partly in composing poems.

In 1736, the fame of him as a rising man had grown so great and spread so far that George II of England, as Elector of Hanover, possibly instigated by Hans Sloane, created for him and offered to him a Chair of Anatomy, Botany and Medicine, in the University of Göttingen. Haller accepted the offer, and here, at Göttingen, for seventeen years he laboured, making physiology the chief duty of the Chair. Here he carried out the most important of his inquiries and gathered together the material for most of his literary work.

He received several tempting offers to accept office in other Universities, in Oxford, Berlin and elsewhere. These he refused; but in 1753 feeling that the increase of years, aided by the climate of Göttingen, was telling upon his health, and he had never been robust, he withdrew to his native city Bern, there to spend the rest of his days in leisurely retirement.

Here or in some neighbouring part of Switzerland he lived for nearly a quarter of a century, refusing to be tempted back to Göttingen or to go elsewhere, taking his part in municipal and other duties, completing his *Elementa* and his other works of compilation or exposition, giving finishing touches to experimental inquiries, and, by way of relaxation, continuing his botanical studies and composing poems and literary essays. Disease however got increasing hold of him, severe pain led him to the constant use of opium, and his medical friend having in 1776 foretold that his death would take place in the following year, he made good the prophecy by quietly passing away on Dec. 12, 1777. He died, true to the errand of his life, with his finger on his pulse, his last words to the friend at his bedside being "The artery no longer beats."

I do not propose now to speak of Haller's many and varied original inquiries, or of the gains which came to physiology thereby. He put his hand to the solution of many questions spread over nearly the whole of physiology; and in the preface to the sixth volume of the *Elementa* he gives a list of what he claims as some of his own discoveries. Of the highest importance were his researches on the mechanics of respiration, on the formation of bone, and on the development of the embryo; the latter indeed stands out as the most conspicuous piece of work on this subject between Malpighi and von Baer, though marred by the theoretical speculations attached to it. Of what is perhaps his greatest work, the establishment of the doctrine of muscular irritability, I shall have occasion to speak in detail in a succeeding lecture. For the present I wish to speak of him as an expositor only. When we turn from any of the preceding writers on physiology, from any one of those whom I have mentioned in the foregoing lectures, and open the pages of Haller's *Elementa*, we feel that we have passed into modern times. Save for the strangeness of much of the nomenclature, and for no small deficiencies in all that relates to the chemical changes of the body, we seem to be reading a modern text-book, a modern text-book of the most laborious and exhaustive kind. Haller passes in review all the phenomena of the body. In dealing with each division of physiology he carefully describes the anatomical basis, including the data of minute structure, physical properties, and chemical composition so far as these were then known. He then states the observations which have been made, and in respect to each question as it arises explains the several views which have been put forward, giving minute and full references to all the authors quoted. And he finally delivers a reasoned critical judgment, expounding the conclusion which may be arrived at, but not omitting to state plainly when necessary the limitations which the lack of adequate evidence places on forming a decided judgment. He carefully recounts and as carefully criticizes all the knowledge which can be gleaned about any question. If he feels unable to come to a decided conclusion he candidly says so. He always strives to be as exact and as clear as possible; conspicuous is the absence from his writings of loose expressions and ill-defined general views such as abound in so many of his predecessors. We may take any part of his great work as a trustworthy account of the knowledge of the time with regard to the questions therein treated.

The following is a brief sketch of the exposition which he gives of digestion. According to him saliva is neither acid nor alkaline; and so far from attributing to it the great virtues claimed for it by Sylvius and Stahl, he seems to regard its great use as being that of softening the food and helping deglutition. In the stomach he recognizes the importance of the tunica villosa, consisting of glands which, very obvious in birds, are not so evident in man; but he thinks that these glands furnish the mucus of the stomach only, the true gastric juice, succus gastricus, ventriculi succus, being secreted by the arteries. The more exact knowledge of nervous action, which, owing largely to his own labours, had been gathered in since Boerhaave's days, led him to discard the idea that a nervous fluid, oozing from the endings of the nerves, intervenes in gastric digestion.

Dwelling on the difficulty of obtaining gastric juice in a pure condition, noting that acidity is often a token of the

onset, and alkalinity of the advance of putrefaction, he concludes that pure gastric juice is neither acid nor alkaline; and
while speaking of it as a macerating liquor which softens and
dissolves the food, he refuses to regard it as a ferment. It is
not a corrosive liquid, as are many acids, and though it may
be at times acid, the acidity is a token of the degeneration of
the digested food, not of digestion itself, which "imparts to
"the food a wholesome animal nature," *i.e.* gives it the
beginning of vitality; and the characteristic of living animal
tissues is, he urges, alkalinity rather than acidity.

Trituration he regards as a useful aid, especially where
hard grains form a part of food, as in that of birds, but only
an aid. "They have done well who have brought back to its
"proper mediocrity the power of trituration so immensely
"exaggerated."

His account of bile shews how much advance had taken
place, through repeated quiet work, in the preceding years.
Bile he insists is not as some have thought a mere excrement.
Retained for a while and slightly altered during its stay in
but not formed by the gall-bladder, secreted on the contrary
by the substance of the liver, partly perhaps from the blood
supplied by the hepatic artery but mainly from that of the
vena porta, bile is a fluid viscid and bitter but not acid, and
indeed not alkaline, a fluid which as all know has the power
of dissolving fat and so acts on a mixture of oil and water
as to form out of them an emulsion; it thus dissolves all the
food into the homogeneous magma which is called chyle. If,
he says, you ligature the duodenum just above the entrance
of the bile duct, you will find the food above the ligature in
the form of grey lumps, below the ligature in the form of a
whitish homogeneous mass. He adds the notable remark that
bile must have some other function than that just described;
for animals deprived of their gall-bladder very rapidly perish,
the exact cause of their death not being clear.

Turning to the pancreas, after remarking that the exaggerated views of Sylvius and De Graaf had long ago been
refuted by Brunner, he insists on the importance of the fact
that its duct opens into the intestine in common with the bile
duct. "All which things being considered, a part at least of

"the usefulness of pancreatic juice will be to dilute and soften
"the cystic juice * * * so that this mixes better with the food.
"Whence you may explain the hunger of the animals from
"which the pancreas has been removed, attributing it to the
"reflux of a sharper bile into the stomach." And he ends with
this saying, prophetic of the work of Bernard a hundred years
later, "There may be other functions of the liquid not as yet
"well known to us." Of the intestinal juice and of the other
later changes taking place along the alimentary canal, he says
nothing to which I need call attention; he seems to think that
the chief event taking place in the intestines is the separation
and absorption of the nutritive constituents, prepared for this
by the action of the stomach and the bile.

It will not have escaped attention that the effect of the
labours of nearly the whole of the seventeenth century and of
the eighteenth century up to Haller's time was on the whole
to depreciate the work of the stomach. In van Helmont's eyes
the stomach was the great digestive organ, and the acidity
of the gastric juice was its strong hand. Succeeding writers
like Sylvius and Stahl insisted on the greater importance of
other juices, and almost all of them, even those who attributed
considerable potency to the gastric juice, denied or at least
doubted its acidity. But the avatar of the gastric juice was
beginning even while Haller was writing his great work.

René Antoine Ferchault de Reaumur stands out as one of
the most striking men of science of the eighteenth century,
and indeed, in some respects, of all time. Born in 1683 at
Rochelle in France, he was educated for the profession of the
law; but possessed of an ample fortune he was under no need
to follow that or any other bread-winning career. Removing
to Paris at the beginning of the eighteenth century, he used
the opportunities which his abundant means afforded him to
carry out many and varied scientific investigations. Of most
of these I have no occasion to speak here. I need not dwell
on his labours in connection with the manufacture of steel.
I need not speak of the thermometer which bears his name,
and which he invented in 1731. Nor shall I here even discuss
his great work on Insects, published during the years 1734–
1742, though this contains much of physiological interest. I

must content myself with pointing out the important results embodied in his treatises on the Digestion of Birds (Sur la Digestion des Oiseaux) which appeared in the 'Memoirs of the Academy of Science of Paris' in 1752.

The problem which he put before himself in this research was:—Are the changes which the food undergoes in the stomach to be regarded as the results of mere trituration, or of a sort of putrefaction, or are they those of solution, effected in some way or other by means of the gastric juice secreted by the stomach? Having in his possession a Kite he took advantage of its well-known habit of rejecting from its stomach things swallowed, such as feathers, which it could not digest. He made use of small metal tubes open at both ends, save that each end was secured with a grating made of threads or fine wire. He gave the Kite some of these tubes, filled with pieces of meat, and he found that when they were rejected the meat had been partially dissolved, but exhibited no odour or other signs of putrefaction. Small fragments of bone similarly introduced into the stomach in metal tubes were also found to be dissolved. The pieces of bone were only partially dissolved, but by giving the same pieces of bone a second and a third time in the same way he found that at last they were almost completely dissolved. But while meat and bone were thus dissolved, vegetable grains or flour similarly exposed in tubes to the action of the stomach seemed to be little altered. He further observed that the tubes when rejected were more or less filled with a yellowish, somewhat opalescent fluid, which to the taste was salt and bitter. Obviously it was this fluid which dissolved the meat and bone. And he put to himself the question, "What then is this liquid "which acts on meat and on bone in some such way as *l'eau* "*régale* acts on gold, but has not the same power over starch "(farina) that *l'eau régale* has over silver? To which of the "solvents which chemistry offers us can this liquid be com- "pared?"

To answer this question he filled his tubes with small pieces of sponge, from which, when rejected, he squeezed out the fluid which they had imbibed. In this way he obtained a quantity, on one occasion 63 grains, of an opalescent fluid, salt to the taste rather than sour, a fluid "which turned blue "paper red." By help of this contrivance he was the first to obtain gastric juice in an approximately pure condition.

With this fluid he attempted to digest *in vitro*. He exposed pieces of meat to the action of it at 32° R. for 24 hours, using similar pieces of meat placed in simple water as a control. His first experiment was wholly a failure. In a second experiment while the control putrefied, the meat in the gastric juice though not very much dissolved was hardly at all putrefied. Digestion therefore was not putrefaction but something actually opposed to that process.

At this stage unfortunately his Kite died and his experiments were stopped.

He continued his investigations, making use of other animals. He gave to a dog some bones, and also some of his tubes containing meat. On killing the dog 24 hours afterwards, he found the bones not crushed but partly dissolved and much altered; the meat in the tubes also was much dissolved though the tubes themselves were hardly or not at all distorted, and therefore had not been crushed. Some further experiments in which he made sheep swallow tubes filled some with chopped green herbs, others with chopped hay, and examined the contents of the tubes by killing the animal and finding them in the paunch 14 hours afterwards, or by waiting until they had been voided, gave dubious or rather negative results. The contents of the tubes were not greatly altered.

Reaumur's investigation left much still to be ascertained; nevertheless he established by direct experiment that the fluid in the stomach, the gastric juice, had a distinct solvent power, that it dissolved various constituents of food, and did so not by inducing or favouring putrefaction, but by some process which was antagonistic to putrefaction. And he arrived at his results by the employment of a wholly new method.

Though his results attracted attention and are referred to by Haller in his *Elementa*, no one for some time followed his line of investigation or adopted his methods. We have to wait for more than a quarter of a century before any fresh real addition to our knowledge of digestion took place. And for this physiology went back once more to Italy.

In the year 1729 there was born at Scandiano near Reggio in Southern Italy Lazaro Spallanzani, the son of a distinguished advocate. He received a very liberal education in letters, being intended by his father for the profession of law, but Vallisnieri, then Professor at Padua, persuaded the father to allow the son to follow in his studies the bent of his mind, which was clearly towards natural science and especially natural history. The celebrated Laura Bassi, then holding, though a woman, the Chair of Mathematics at Bologna, was his cousin; he studied under her and her teaching seems to have confirmed his love for science. In 1754 he became 'Professor of Logic, Mathematics and Greek at Reggio, but in 1760 was transferred to Modena to fill the Chair of Natural History. In 1768, the Empress Maria Theresa, who was developing and indeed re-establishing the University of Pavia, invited him to become professor there of natural history; and he accepted the offer. He was pressed in 1785 on the death of Vallisnieri to succeed that great naturalist in the Chair of Natural History in the University of Padua; but he refused, taking advantage however of the invitation to obtain leave for a long travel in Turkey. By specimens obtained in this and in his other many travels he enriched the museum of the University of Pavia, to which he remained devoted. He died in that city on Feb. 3, 1799. In the course of his education before his appointment at Reggio he had taken orders in the Church, and is frequently spoken of as the Abbé Spallanzani; but nearly the whole of his energy was thrown into the investigation of problems of natural history. His works on Reproduction brought him great fame; his contributions to the physiology of the circulation were considerable; he travelled much and worked at geological problems; and just before his death he carried out researches on respiration in which he made a notable addition to that part of physiology for which Lavoisier had just done so much. But here I wish to speak only of his contributions to the physiology of digestion, his first memoir on which was published in 1777, the year of Haller's death, others following in the succeeding years.

He took up again Reaumur's method, and most of his results were gained by it, though he also adopted other methods. Finding the knowledge of the subject almost in the condition in which Reaumur had left it, he was able by his numerous experiments, aided by the improvements in chemistry since Reaumur's time, to make a great advance over his French predecessor.

He experimented with all kinds of animals (and he was it may be noted not a mere physiologist but a naturalist, one who studied animals (and plants) from various points of view), fishes, frogs, newts, serpents, birds of various kinds, sheep, oxen, horses, cats, dogs, and lastly himself. He at least ran no risk of going astray by making deductions based on results gained with one kind of animal only.

He employed largely, as I have said, Reaumur's method. He made use of metal tubes, closed by a grating at each end; but in order to allow the freer entrance of fluid he also made perforations in the walls. Sometimes he used hollow spheres made of two hemispheres screwed together, the walls being freely perforated. These tubes or spheres he filled with pieces of meat, bread or bone, or grains of wheat and the like. He recovered them in the case of carnivorous birds through their being rejected by the mouth; in the case of other animals he opened the stomach after the lapse of a given time.

He also made animals swallow pieces of meat or the like, so attached to threads or wires that he could after a while withdraw them from the stomach.

On himself he experimented by swallowing small linen bags containing meat, bread, etc. and examining the contents after they had been voided per anum. Greatly daring he swallowed perforated tubes, made not of metal but wood; and these he successfully recovered without suffering any harm.

He obtained what he speaks of as gastric juice by making animals swallow on an empty stomach tubes containing sponges. On recovering the tubes he found that the sponges had imbibed a considerable quantity of fluid, which he squeezed out. From himself he obtained gastric juice by making himself vomit on an empty stomach before breakfast;

but this mode of experimentation was he says so disagreeable that after two trials he gave it up.

The action of the gastric juice so obtained he tested on various articles of food *in vitro*, exposing tubes containing the juice and food to warmth either by keeping them in his own armpit for two or three days, or by placing them in a stove, and always using as a control the same food covered with simple water.

By a very large number of experiments carried on in these various ways he confirmed and greatly extended Reaumur's results. He found that in all animals food is in the living stomach dissolved "into the pultaceous mass called chyme" by the juice to whose action it is there subjected; and that this juice is a solvent of all kinds of food, animal and vegetable, bone included, though some things or parts are more soluble than others. He found that the juice was more active on divided parts, such as crushed grains, or broken bones, than on whole solid parts, such as whole bones, or whole grains; from this he concluded that "trituration is merely a "preparation for solution and does not itself constitute the "digestive process." He was led by his numerous experiments to the same conclusion as Reaumur, that while gastric juice was a solvent of all kinds of food, the juice of this or that animal was more specially active on the natural food of the animal, that the juice of the herbivorous animal for instance was more active on vegetable food. Recalling Reaumur's experiment of giving green plants or hay to sheep in tubes, he repeated the experiment and obtained at first similar negative results, even in the case of tubes which had passed into the fourth stomach. But, remembering that the sheep always ruminated, and prepared its food for solution by prolonged mastication, he repeated the experiment with the variation that he carefully masticated the food, herbs or hay, before he introduced it into the tubes. He then found that the contents of the tubes were largely dissolved. He concluded that mastication with the attendant admixture of saliva was, like the trituration in the muscular stomachs, a preparation for the solvent action of the gastric juice.

His experiments with gastric juice removed from the living stomach and made to act on food *in vitro* fully confirmed the results obtained in the living stomach itself. Food of very various kinds thus exposed to the action of gastric juice was dissolved and did not putrefy, whereas the same food sub-jected to the action of simple water soon putrefied. Solution *in vitro* was however never so rapid or complete as in the living stomach. Thinking that this might be due to the fact that in the experiment out of the body the gastric juice is not renewed as it is in the living stomach, he endeavoured to imitate the natural process by allowing his gastric juice to fall drop by drop on, and to run away drop by drop from, pieces of meat and bread. He now found that "solution took place with ex-"ceeding speed." He observed that in all cases heat favoured solution; indeed in warm-blooded animals a certain high temperature seemed to him necessary, though cold-blooded animals did not need this.

It was clear from his experiments that gastric juice was a powerful solvent of all kinds of food. The question now arose, What was the nature of this solvent power? "It remains," says he, "to be inquired whether this function is connected "with a principle of acidity, as some suppose, or of putre-"faction according to others."

The supposition of putrefaction was soon disposed of; so far from producing or even assisting putrefaction, the gastric juice was actually opposed to putrefaction; meat which in simple water readily putrefied in the warm, remained sweet in gastric juice kept equally warm; the gastric juice even destroyed the putridity of putrid meat.

Putrefaction in Spallanzani's time, as of old, was regarded as one of the modes of fermentation; but by his time the general ideas about fermentation had become more clearly defined. It was no longer confounded with the effervescence due to mere chemical action. "There are," says Spallanzani, "three kinds of fermentation: the vinous or sweet, the "acetous, and the putrid." The action of the gastric juice was not a putrid fermentation; could it be one of the other two? He was inclined to believe that the action could not be considered as any kind of fermentation at all, because bubbles of air formed a necessary feature of every fermentation in a liquid, and solution by gastric juice could and generally did take place without any bubbles of gas being formed. The action certainly was not a vinous fermentation, since neither gas nor alcohol was formed. Could it be of the nature of acetous fermentation? In discussing this Spallanzani enters on the question whether gastric juice is acid.

It will be remembered that though van Helmont had put in the foreground the acid nature of the digestive fermentation taking place in the stomach, succeeding writers had denied this and did so as time went on with increasing assuredness, though Spallanzani as we have just seen referred to its being still maintained by some. Spallanzani's results led him to agree with the dominant view. It may here be remarked that when Spallanzani speaks of gastric juice he means something which he regards as a mixed fluid. The juice which he squeezed out of the sponges contained in the tubes recovered from the stomach he describes as "a transparent "yellow fluid which gave very little sediment on standing, "which had a taste intermediate between bitter and salt, "which was not very volatile and which certainly contained "no inflammable components." When on the other hand he opened the stomach of dogs and examined the liquid which oozed out from the surface of the lining mucous membrane, he found that this was "colourless, insipid and very thin," thus contrasting with that which is generally found in the interior of the cavity of the stomach when opened, this being yellow, bitter and somewhat gelatinous, like the material imbibed by the sponges in the tube. Hence he inferred that what he called gastric juice was a mixture consisting of the above proper secretion of the stomach, "thin, colourless and "insipid," together with saliva, juice secreted by the glands of the oesophagus, bile and possibly pancreatic juice; bile seemed to be always present in his specimens of gastric juice and to this he attributed the bitter taste. The activity of this mixed juice was probably due to the constituent supplied by the stomach itself, for when he introduced into birds, such as crows, two pieces of meat fastened on a wire so that the lower one reached the stomach but the upper remained in the oesophagus, the former was much more readily dissolved than the latter; similarly when he introduced a long rod of meat reaching through the oesophagus into the stomach, this was much corroded at the end which reached into the stomach, but very little above. But he did not follow up the investigation into the properties of pure gastric juice, and contented himself with the results obtained from the mixed contents of the stomach.

He repeatedly tried to obtain evidence of the presence of acids in this mixed gastric juice but failed to obtain anything which could satisfy him. Though he observed that shells and corals were corroded in the stomach of birds, he could not find any clear indication of acidity in the stomach other than that which was due to the tendency of food to turn sour; and this, says he, is an abnormal and not a healthy condition.

"I repeatedly dropped gastric juice upon salt of *tartar per* "*deliquium* and into the nitrous and marine acids without "ever perceiving any change of colour, any motion or "effervescence; whence I am obliged to infer that the gastric "juice is neither acid nor alkaline, but neutral." His own gastric juice, obtained as we have seen by vomiting, he also found to be neutral; and he is confirmed in his belief that acidity of the gastric juice is something abnormal by the reflection that regurgitation of sour material from the stomach into the mouth only occurs when digestion has gone wrong; and he quotes his own experience of acid fluid coming up into his mouth after a too great indulgence in strawberries and white wine, which had obviously disagreed with him.

It will be interesting to quote here what is perhaps the earliest analysis of gastric juice. Spallanzani asked his colleague and friend, Scopoli, Professor of Chemistry at Pavia, to examine for him the gastric juice which he had obtained from crows by his sponges and tubes. This is what the chemist reports: "The fluid contains first pure water, "secondly a saponaceous and gelatinous animal substance, "thirdly sal ammoniac, and fourthly an earthy matter like "that which exists in all animal fluids. It precipitates silver "from nitrous acid and forms luna cornea. This phenomenon

"might induce us to suppose that common salt exists in the
"gastric juice; but the salt contained in this fluid is not
"common salt, but sal ammoniac."

Spallanzani thus came to the conclusion that gastric juice
is not acid, though he asked himself the question whether
since it curdled milk it might not contain "an acid in some
"latent form."

Since then gastric juice was not acid, solution of food by
its means could not be of the nature of acetous fermentation
any more than it was of the nature of vinous or putrid fermentation. It was not any of the known forms of fermentation;
it was not a fermentation at all.

We thus owe to Spallanzani, after Reaumur, the definite
experimental proof of the solvent power of gastric juice over
various constituents of food. But he was unable to go beyond
this, because he failed to recognize its acid character; he
could only say that the action was not a fermentation in the
then usual sense of that word; he could not explain how this
apparently neutral fluid possessed these solvent powers. We
may wonder how so acute an observer missed the acidity of
gastric juice. We may partly explain this by the fact that he
confined his tests for acidity to the gastric juice which he had
obtained from fasting stomachs, including that obtained from
himself, and apparently did not test the juice which had
actually digested the material contained in his tubes. Still
in some or other of his almost innumerable experiments he
must, we might fancy, have come upon evidences of acidity
so distinct that he could not overlook it. Possibly even he,
accurate and unbiased observer as he certainly was, may
have been misled by preconceived opinion; when he came
upon acidity he regarded it as something abnormal.

Be it as it may, by Spallanzani's labours, the fact of the
solvent power of gastric juice as a power which was *sui generis*,
the solution effected by which was not the solution of putrefaction, or of any other known form of fermentation such
as might occur under various circumstances, whether within
or outside the stomach, became an established fact, a definite
addition, never afterwards taken away, to our knowledge of
digestion.

I ought to add that in an Inaugural Dissertation which appeared in the same year as Spallanzani's first memoir, namely in 1777, Stevens of Edinburgh, adopting Reaumur's methods, had arrived at results similar to those of the French and Italian inquirers. Taking advantage "of a man of weak "understanding who gained a miserable livelihood by swallow-"ing stones for the amusement of the common people," Stevens made him swallow silver perforated spheres con-taining pieces of food, animal and vegetable, raw and cooked and including bone; he found on examining the spheres, when after some forty-eight hours they were voided, that the food was for the most part dissolved; whole grains however of wheat, peas, etc. were but little changed. He continued his experiments on dogs, making them swallow similar spheres, killing them after a variable number of hours and opening their stomachs. He repeated the experiments on sheep and oxen, and found that while these digested readily vegetables, hay and herbs, their stomachs had little action on animal food. He then obtained 'pure gastric fluid' from the stomach of a dog killed after a fast of sixteen hours, and found that this fluid at a temperature of 102–104° Fahr. readily dissolved cooked meat, without any putrefaction and without any development of air bubbles. He thus came with Spallanzani to the conclusion that digestion "is not the effect of heat, "trituration, putrefaction or fermentation alone, but of a "powerful solvent secreted by the coats of the stomach which "converts the aliment into a fluid resembling the blood." He adds, "It is probable that every species of animal has its "peculiar gastric liquor capable of dissolving certain sub-"stances only." The conclusions are almost identical with those of Spallanzani, but did not attract so much attention as did those of the Italian philosopher.

About the time that Spallanzani was conducting his re-searches on digestion, the great English surgeon John Hunter was also turning his attention to the same subject. In 1772 he published in the *Philosophical Transactions* a paper 'On the Digestion of the Stomach after Death'; and his *Obser-vations on Certain Parts of the Animal Economy*, the first edition of which appeared in 1786, contains a memoir entitled

'Observations on Digestion.' In the latter publication Hunter went out of his way not only to say that a statement by Reaumur which he quotes "is to be set down as a piece "of anatomical ignorance," but also to criticize severely several particular experiments of Spallanzani as well as his general method of inquiry. He complained of Spallanzani as being deficient in anatomical knowledge, and in that "like "all mere experiment-makers, he is not satisfied even with "those which are clear and decisive, but multiplies them most "unnecessarily." He explained how in his view experiments ought to be conducted and adds that "if Spallanzani had "employed half his time in this way * * * he had employed "his time much better than in making experiments without "end." This rude and disdainful criticism Spallanzani answered and adequately rebuked in a dignified manner in a letter published in 1788. One cannot help suspecting that the tone of Hunter's remarks was in part at least due to a want of sympathy between Spallanzani's general views and his own. For Spallanzani was eminently free from all vitalistic tendencies. On the other hand, to understand Hunter's views it must be borne in mind that he distinctly belonged to the school of Stahl though he replaced the phrase 'sensitive soul' by that of 'vital principle.'

"An animal substance," says he, "when joined with the "living principle, cannot undergo any change in its properties "but as an animal; this principle always acting and preserving "the substance possessed of it from dissolution, and from "being changed according to the natural changes which other "substances undergo." The doctrine here laid down is, it will be observed, almost identical with that of Stahl.

In his first paper Hunter states that "the appearances of "the stomach found to be digested after death shew that "digestion neither depends on a mechanical power, nor con-"tractions of the stomach, nor on heat, but on something "secreted in the coats of the stomach, and thrown into its "cavity, which there animalizes the food or assimilates it to "the nature of blood." The instances of the stomach digesting itself interested him, because he maintained that "animals or "parts of animals, possessed of the living principle, when

"taken into the stomach, are not in the least affected by the
"powers of that viscus, so long as the animal principle re-
"mains." And he explained the auto-digestion as due to the
walls of the stomach ceasing to be alive and becoming subject
to the power still remaining in the gastric juice which they
had themselves secreted.

Hunter is very clear that digestion is not fermentation.
He speaks of the vinous and acetous fermentation to which
vegetable substances are prone and of the putrefactive fermentation to which animal substances are subject. And he
argues as follows:—"It may be admitted as an axiom that
"two processes cannot go on at the same time in the same
"part of any substance; therefore neither vegetable nor
"animal substances can undergo their spontaneous changes
"while in the act of being digested, it being a process superior
"in power to that of fermentation. * * * The gastric juice
"therefore preserves vegetables from running into fermenta-
"tion and animal substances from putrefaction; not from any
"antiseptic quality in the juice, but, by making them go
"through another process, preventing the spontaneous change
"from taking place."

And he develops his view more fully as follows: "The
"process of digestion differs from every other natural opera-
"tion in the change it produces on different bodies; yet it is
"by no means fermentation, though it may resemble it. For
"fermentation, a spontaneous process, is that natural suc-
"cession of changes by which vegetable and animal matter
"is reduced to earth; therefore must be widely different from
"digestion which converts both animal and vegetable sub-
"stances into chyle, in the formation of which there cannot
"be a decomposition similar to fermentation.

"Digestion is likewise very different from chemical solution,
"which is only a union of bodies by elective attraction. But
"digestion is an assimilating process; and in this respect is
"somewhat similar in its action to that excited by morbid
"poisons. It is a species of generation, two substances making
"a third; but the curious circumstance is its converting both
"vegetable and animal matter into the same kind of substance
"or compound, which no chemical process can effect. The

"chyle is compounded of the gastric juice and digestible
"substances when perfectly converted; and it is probable that
"the quantity of gastric juice may be nearly equal to that
"part of the food which is really changed into chyle."

Hunter's views here, it will be seen, are very similar to
those of Spallanzani, though modified by the vitalistic Stahlian
conceptions in which the latter did not share. In one respect
Hunter went beyond Spallanzani; he was, at least at one time,
inclined to attach importance to the acidity of gastric juice.
In 1772 he says: "In all the animals, whether carnivorous or
"not, upon which I made experiments to discover whether or
"not there was an acid in the stomach (and I tried this in a
"great variety), I constantly found that there was an acid,
"though not a strong one, in the juices contained in that
"viscus in a natural state." But in his later paper he is led
to think that "it is only formed occasionally. Whether the
"stomach has the power of immediately secreting this acid,
"or first secretes a sugar which afterwards becomes acid, is
"not easily ascertained." He is inclined towards the latter
view, especially since in the stomach of the calf before birth
no acid can be found. And indeed the eighteenth century
passed wholly away before the 'acid ferment' on which van
Helmont had, in the early years of the seventeenth century,
laid such great stress was rightly appreciated. For the observation of Carminati who, following close after Spallanzani,
in 1785 found the clue to the problem of the acidity of gastric
juice, by shewing that in carnivora at least the juice though
neutral when the animal is starving, is undoubtedly indeed
strongly acid after it has been fed, fell on barren ground,
and failed to produce the fruit which otherwise it might.

During the two centuries, the seventeenth and the
eighteenth, physiological inquirers, as we have seen, swayed
now in one direction, by views of chemical fermentation or
effervescence, now in another direction by views of mechanical
trituration, had come in the end to the conclusion that digestion
was in the main a process of solution of a peculiar character
begun and chiefly carried out in the stomach though assisted
by minor subsequent changes taking place along the intestines.
They who were under the influence of the Stahlian vitalistic

doctrines, and these were perhaps the more numerous, held the change to be the commencement of, to be the first step in, the conversion of dead food into living flesh and blood, and spoke of it as an animalization. They who were not of that school were content to speak of it as a change differing from ordinary chemical change, without being able to define its exact characters. It was left for the nineteenth century to throw a new light on the nature of the gastric changes and at the same time to shew that what took place in the stomach was not the whole of digestion, but only the first of a series of profound changes taking place along nearly the whole length of the alimentary canal.

LECTURE IX

THE RISE OF THE MODERN DOCTRINES OF RESPIRATION. BLACK, PRIESTLEY, LAVOISIER

WE have seen in a preceding lecture how far John Mayow went in the knowledge of the chemistry of breathing. He wrote in the third quarter of the seventeenth century; and by the end of the century his views had well-nigh passed away from men's minds. Some writers it is true still spoke of 'nitrous particles' playing a part in breathing, but the ideas which were thus put forth were more akin to the loose notions which we have seen Sylvius held, than to the clear and definite conception of Mayow. We have dwelt, in a preceding lecture, on the chemical activity of Stahl, and, looking at the matter in the light of our present knowledge, it seems difficult to understand how it was that the foremost chemist of the early years of the eighteenth century, who busied himself especially with the nature of combustion and with the theory of phlogiston, did not put forward some striking chemical theory of breathing. That he did not do so seems to have been due to the way in which his mind was influenced by views which he had adopted concerning the physical and mechanical effects of the flow of blood through the capillaries.

Stahl taught that the most important fact about the circulation of the blood was the passage through the capillaries, the "transpression of the blood through the spongy, porous "and exceedingly soft tissues of the body, by which doubtless "it is kept constantly in a proper state of fluidity so that it "may remain not only suited for its perpetual circuit but also "fitted for the due separation during that very circuit of the "matters which have to be discharged from its midst."

He insisted that two things have to be borne in mind in relation to this "transpulsion through the soft porous tissues. "The first is the business of the vital tonic movement, which "takes place and is developed in an independent manner, "quite apart from our will and consciousness. By means of "this the porous structures at one time being more con-"stricted and compact, admit the blood more sparingly, and "at another time being relaxed, give place to a readier and

"fuller passage." This idea of the varying tonicity, of the
varying tonic movement, of the tissues was made by Stahl
the corner-stone of much of his pathology, and exerted a
powerful influence over medical thought for many years.

The second thing on which Stahl insisted as a result of the
'transpulsion' is the warming of the blood. "The second
"point to be noticed is the heating of the blood under, nay
"rather on account of, this same movement of the circulation
"at once pulsatory and tonic, and of the special intensity of
"each of these two kinds of movement." The heating, he
says, is simply the mechanical effect of the friction developed
during the passage. "Here again we ought to bear in mind
"the purely mechanical nature of the whole action. That is
"to say, this heating does not depend on any foreign par-
"ticular kind of matter (except alone the special chemical
"constitution of the blood itself), but solely and simply on
"the movement and on its greater or less intensity, the
"variations of which are dependent on the one hand on the
"impetus itself of the impulse, and on the other hand on the
"tonic rigidity of the tissues according as these are con-
"stricted or relaxed."

Stahl thus deliberately rejects the view that the heat of
the blood and so of the body is due to chemical action; he
regards it as solely and simply a mechanical effect. And this
conception of the origin of animal heat determined his view
of the function of breathing. According to him, the purpose
of the movements of the chest and of the lungs is to regulate
and facilitate the passage of the blood through the pulmonary
blood vessels, and he discusses at length how the rhythmic
movement, the alternate expansion and contraction of the
chest affects the condition of blood vessels in the lungs, and
so the flow through them. And he takes credit to himself
for being the first to shew that so far from breathing having
a cooling effect on the blood, the friction engendered by the
passage of blood through the lungs is one of the chief sources
of the heat of the body.

Thus the great chemist of the day was, by the influence of
a theory, led away from the true solution of one of the most
conspicuous chemical problems of physiology. And this was

the case, although he had put his foot on the right path. Discussing the uses of air, he dwells briefly on the question whether something may not in inspiration be given up to the blood, just as in expiration there is, as he admits, a "transpiration of aquosity in the form of vapour"; but he concludes that any such entrance is of little moment; and he sums up as follows:

"As however it is quite evident that air thus takes part in "and contributes to this whole business of breathing in no "other than a formal manner, as the phrase is" (that is in a mechanical manner), "so, as to whether, where and how it may "seem to add something in the way of mere matter, we have "already made a remark or two. Meanwhile it is wholly clear, "from every point of view, that that something is neither "great in quantity nor dense in quality, nor indeed anything "different from the true nature of atmospheric air, which it "must necessarily be if breathing supplied any kind of spirit "to the blood. If it be anything it must be something much "more simple, namely a certain principle called phlogiston. "Nevertheless in respect even to this, doubts against it of no "less weight than arguments in favour of it present them- "selves. For this principle does not abound in the air in "sufficient quantity to be able at each breath to supply and "add to the blood an amount of itself of any moment. This "is *a posteriori* clear from the fact that only a very little of "this matter of phlogiston can be received into even a large "quantity of air, even in a place where it is sufficiently "collected in it, as when inflammable things are burnt. How- "ever these things may be, these considerations, interesting "perhaps to the curious, add absolutely nothing to medical "practice; and it is not meet to waste any more time upon "them."

Thus the great exponent of the chemistry of his time, and especially of the chemistry of combustion, touched lightly the key to one of the most important of the chemical problems of the living body, and having touched it, deliberately drew his hand away.

We naturally turn from Stahl to learn the views of the other great chemist of the period, Hermann Boerhaave. We

must remember that the two were men of very unlike character. Stahl was an investigator and an eager promulgator
of new views; Boerhaave, though he did pursue with zeal and
success various experimental inquiries, was in the main an
expositor and an eclectic critic of the views of others. He put
forward no new theories of his own about breathing, and was
content to point out the conclusions which could be drawn
from the various results of other inquirers. In his great work
on the *Elements of Chemistry*, which deservedly became the
text-book of the age, after dwelling at some length on air and
its properties in a manner which shews his profound acquaintance with all the researches of the time, he has a passage
entitled "There is in air a wholly special virtue." In this,
after shewing that all living things stand in need of air, and
after pointing out the effect of air on the colour of blood, in
turning dark blood scarlet, he ends as follows:

"All these things prove that air possesses a certain occult
"virtue which cannot be explained by any of those properties
"of air which have hitherto been investigated. That in this
"virtue the secret food of life lies hidden some chemists have
"asserted. But what it really is, how it acts and what it
"exactly brings about is still obscure. Happy the man who
"will discover it !"

We may recognize in this the sagacious observer groping
round the truth but unable to lay his finger exactly on it.
What were Boerhaave's more detailed teachings concerning
breathing may be inferred from the exposition given by his
illustrious pupil Haller; for Haller in the main followed the
lines of his great master, differing from him chiefly in the
matters which were the subjects of his own original investigations.

In his third volume, which is devoted to respiration, Haller
begins the subject with an account of the thorax and its
contents, and of the actions and uses of the various parts.
Then follows a discussion of the physical properties of air,
its weight and its 'spring.' In the course of this he dwells on
the causes which destroy the 'spring' of air, noting as chief
among these the respiration of animals, and observing that
while this loss of 'spring' seems to be intimately connected

with the fact that animals cannot live in air which is not renewed, the exact cause why they cannot do so is by no means clear. Next, after an exposition of the general phenomena and of the more mechanical problems of respiration, he comes to the use of breathing and asks the question, Why almost all animals stand in need of air? This leads to the question, Whether air enters into and is mixed with the blood in breathing? In respect to this he quotes three leading opinions.

"From the most ancient times it has been a common view "that as air is in nature the cause of almost all movement and "without it fire cannot subsist or charcoal take fire, so also "air enters into the vital humours of animals and provides "in them that which brings about life. Very many are the "authors who have approved of this view, among whom I will "only mention the chief, and of these the more recent, who "have maintained that the very air of the atmosphere itself, "such as we take in by the mouth, reaches the blood. A "different opinion is held by those who have admitted that "only a something reaches the blood from the air, which "something some have spoken of as the more subtle particles "or ether, others again as aereal nitre. A third party have "maintained that the very air itself reaches the blood but "air dissolved in water and deprived of its elastic force so "that it cannot expand or undergo compression."

In discussing these several views Haller naturally dwells upon the corresponding views held as to the use or function of the air or part of the air thus reaching the blood. He speaks of what may be called the physical hypothesis, such as that held by Borelli, which taught that the air, still retaining its elasticity, produced its effect on the blood in a physical manner, by exciting vibrations for instance. He mentions the various forms of the spiritual hypothesis, according to which either an actual vital spirit, or some active particles, spirituous or ethereal, passed from the air into the blood and gave it its vital properties. He adds, "Some indeed while "refusing to admit in plain terms that any actual spirit is "generated out of the air, nevertheless affirm that a vital "entity of some kind is taken up from the air, and indeed "men, wholly opposed to the vitalistic sect" (referring to the passage of Boerhaave quoted above), "have not shrunk from "this view." He next refers to the chemical hypothesis, namely, that some chemical substance, a saline vapour, or an acid volatile salt, or aereal nitre, passed from the air into the blood and produced an effect on the blood through chemical processes; and he places the views of Mayow on the same level as those of the many other chemical authors.

Discussing and rejecting all these various views, giving his reasons for thinking that elastic air does not pass into the blood, and refuting at some length the hypothesis that the inspired air, through being cold, leads to a condensation of the blood in the lungs, Haller warns the reader that the rejection of all these views "does not lead to the conclusion "that in breathing we derive nothing from the air."

He argues that since air exists in such quantity in all the humours of the body and since a ready entrance of air is afforded by the absorbing veinlets surrounding the pulmonary vesicles full of air, air does enter the blood, but "in the lungs "loses its elastic nature and so becomes readily soluble in "water and vapour. Hippocrates counted air as a nutriment "of the body, and since even the most solid parts of the body "contain a great deal of air and give that up when they are "dissolved and reduced to their elements, it is extremely "probable that air plays the part of a cement holding "together the earthy elements."

Such is Haller's account of pulmonary inhalation, and he completes the story by an account of pulmonary exhalation, which he says consists chiefly of water but not mere water, "water impregnated with a volatile fatty exhalation and not "free from saline matter."

The subject of animal heat is so closely connected with respiration that it will be convenient to note here what Haller has to say about this. He expounds in the first place what may be called the chemical theories of animal heat, the fermentation in the heart, as put forward by van Helmont, and the effervescence arising from the meeting of the old used-up blood, spoken of as venous blood, and the fresh acid chyle, as put forward by Sylvius. He merely touches in a very scanty manner only on the more exact chemical view of Mayow. But he goes on to say that "towards the close of the preceding "(seventeenth) century greater attention was paid to the "properties of solid parts, and the importance attached to "chemical causes (such as van Helmont and Sylvius had "brought to the front) somewhat fell off." Hence there came into more general acceptance the physical view that the heat of the body was due to the friction of the blood as it was driven through the blood vessels, the view held as we have just seen by Stahl.

Haller discusses all the various arguments for and against these several views, and concludes as follows:

"So far then it seems most probable that the blood is "certainly warmed by its movement, but it is by no means "clear why it should be thus warmed to a higher degree than "water would be under like circumstances, or why the tem-"perature is never varied beyond certain narrow limits."

I have given this brief sketch of Haller's exposition in order to shew how little advance has been made since the days of the English School of which I spoke in a preceding lecture. Perhaps one ought rather to say how things had gone back, for the lead offered by Mayow as it had been rejected by those coming between him and Haller, so it was rejected by Haller himself.

Meanwhile the first step in the new progress which before long was to be made had been taken, and that in Mayow's country, in England, or rather in Great Britain.

Well known to Haller, though perhaps not fully appreciated by him, were the works of Stephen Hales. This remarkable man did not belong to the medical profession, was not the holder of any medical chair. He was a clergyman, an active, perhaps too active, and zealous parish priest. Born in 1677 at Bekesbourne in Kent, educated at Corpus Christi College in Cambridge, of which he was some time a Fellow, he became perpetual curate or minister at Teddington on the Thames, where he made the acquaintance of Horace Walpole, who however speaks of him 'as a poor, good, primitive creature,' of Pope and others. He was also Rector of Farringdon in Hampshire. He died in 1761. Clergyman as he was, he was devoted to science; he had begun to experiment while at Cambridge "in the elaboratory of Trinity College" which the then Master of Trinity, the great scholar Bentley, anxious to make his College the seat of all kinds of learning, had established; and he continued his researches amid his parish duties at Teddington. He was a sanitary pioneer, being the first to introduce ventilation, an ardent advocate of temperance principles, and one of the founders of a society which afterwards became the present Society of Arts. The Royal Society, of which he was an active Fellow, published his *Statical Essays*, the first volume of which appeared in 1726, the second in 1732. The second volume entitled *Haemastatics* deals chiefly with the mechanics of circulation. He was the first to determine, by actual experiment on the living animal (he used the horse), the pressure of blood on the blood vessels; and the researches recorded in this volume stand out conspicuous as marking the chief advance made in this branch of physiology between Borelli and Poisseuille. The first volume, which treats chiefly of the flow of sap in vegetables, contains an essay with the following title:

"A specimen of an attempt to analyse the air by a great "variety of chymico-statical experiments which shew in how "great a proportion air is wrought into the composition of "animal, vegetable, and mineral substances, and withal "how readily it assumes its former elastic state when, in "the dissolution of those substances it is disengaged from "them."

He calls all gases 'air,' and recognizes air or gas as existing, first in an elastic state, in which the particles repel each other, and secondly in a reduced or fixed state, in which their particles are attracted by the particles of some other substance, *e.g.* sulphureous particles.

I refer to him not because he made any definite special contribution to our knowledge of respiration (though his work had a remarkable practical side through the introduction of ventilation), but because his writings contain the first clear enunciation of the existence of gases in a free and in a combined condition. By clearly stating this principle he exercised a notable influence on other men's researches, and thus powerfully aided the discoveries which were made by others after him. This is what he says:

"Since, then, air is found so manifestly to abound in almost "all natural bodies; since we find it so operative and active a "principle in every chymical operation; since its constituent "parts are of so durable a nature, that the most violent action "of fire or of fermentation cannot induce such an alteration "of its texture as thereby to disqualify it from resuming either "by fire or fermentation its former elastick state;...since then "this is the case, may we not with good reason adopt this "now fixed, now volatile Proteus among the chymical prin-"ciples, and that a very active one, as well as acid sulphur? "notwithstanding it has hitherto been overlooked and re-"jected by chymists, as in no way entitled to that denomina-"tion."

Hales, it will be observed, speaks of air (or gas) as if it were always the same thing. He knew that air had not always the same properties, that sometimes it was inflammable and sometimes not, sometimes good for breathing, sometimes not, but these were instances of varying qualities of the same thing, not of different things. He ignored van Helmont's discovery of a gas which was a different thing from air. But the avatar of the now nearly forgotten van Helmont was soon to come.

In 1754 there appeared a *Dissertatio de humore acido a cibo orto et de magnesia* by one Joseph Black, who, born at Bordeaux in 1728, had been educated at Belfast, Glasgow, and Edinburgh, and who in the year following the appearance of his dissertation was appointed Professor of Chemistry at Glasgow in succession to Cullen. Ten years later he became, again in succession to Cullen, Professor of Chemistry at Edinburgh, where he died in 1799. The Latin dissertation of 1754 appeared in the following year as an English essay, entitled, 'Experiments on Magnesia Alba, Quick-lime, and other Alkaline Substances.'

Stone in the bladder and gravel in the urine were in those days attracting much attention in the medical profession, and the qualities of various alkaline bodies proposed as remedies for them were being much discussed.

According to prevalent ideas, governed by the phlogiston theory of Stahl, lime or chalk became quick-lime, became caustic by taking up phlogiston, and when slacked gave out phlogiston; that is to say lime suffered gain in becoming caustic quick-lime, and caustic quick-lime suffered loss in being slacked and becoming mild.

Black made the notable observation that ordinary or mild lime lost in weight when it was burnt into caustic lime. He further observed that all 'mild' alkalis, lime, magnesia, and the like, when treated with acids, gave off a particular kind of gas or air. When caustic lime by exposure to the air became mild lime, the change, he argued, consisted in the lime taking up from the atmosphere this particular kind of air. "Quick-"lime therefore does not attract air when in its most ordinary "form, but is capable of being joined to one particular species "only, which is dispersed through the atmosphere either in "the shape of an exceedingly subtle powder, or more probably "in that of an elastic fluid. To this I have given the name of "'fixed air.'"

Moreover when mild lime was burned and so became caustic lime, this same fixed air was given off. It was the loss of this fixed air which accounted for the loss of weight when mild lime was burned into quick-lime. In fact the mild alkalis were compounds of caustic alkalis with fixed air.

This discovery of Black really entailed the destruction of the phlogiston theory, but that theory had established itself in the minds of men of the time far too firmly to be driven off at the first assault.

Black moreover made another discovery. Using as a test for the presence of fixed air the fact that it, when driven through a clear solution of lime water, i.e. a solution of caustic lime, caused a precipitation, in consequence of its combining with the caustic lime and converting it into mild lime, he was able to prove that fixed air was given off in fermentation, was a product of the burning of charcoal and was present in expired air.

He thus rediscovered the gas which van Helmont had discovered more than a hundred years before. This is what he says, writing some years afterwards in his *Treatise of Chemistry*:

"I fully intended to make this air (fixed air) the subject of
"serious study....In the same year, however, in which my first
"account of these experiments (on magnesia, etc.) was pub-
"lished, namely 1757 (*sic*), I had discovered that this par-
"ticular kind of air, attracted by alkaline substances, is
"deadly to all animals that breathe it by the mouth and
"nostrils together; but that if the nostrils were kept shut I
"was led to think that it might be breathed with safety. I
"found for example that when sparrows died in it in ten or
"eleven seconds, they woud live in it for three or four minutes
"when the nostrils were shut by melted suet. And I con-
"vinced myself that the change produced on wholesome air
"by breathing it consisted chiefly, if not solely, in the con-
"version of part of it into fixed air. For I found, that by
"blowing through a pipe into lime water, or a solution of
"caustic alkali, the lime was precipitated, and the alkali was
"rendered mild. I was partly led to these experiments by
"some observations of Dr Hales, in which he says, that
"breathing through diaphragms of cloth dipped in alkaline
"solution made the air last longer for the purposes of life.

"In the same year I found that fixed air is the chief part
"of the elastic matter which is formed in liquids in the vinous
"fermentation. Van Helmont had indeed said this, and it was
"to this that he first gave the name *gas silvestre*. It could
"not long be unknown to those occupied in brewing or making
"wines. But it was at random that he said it was the same
"with that of the Grotto del Cane in Italy (but he supposed
"the identity, because both are deadly), for he had examined
"neither of them chemically, nor did he know that it was the
"air disengaged in the effervescence of alkaline substances
"with acids. I convinced myself of the fact by going to a
"brewhouse with two phials, one filled with distilled water,
"and the other with lime water. I emptied the first into a
"vat of wort fermenting briskly, holding the mouth of the
"phial close to the surface of the wort. I then poured some
"of the lime water into it, shut it with my finger, and shook
"it. The lime water became turbid immediately.

"Van Helmont says that the *dunste* or deadly vapour of
"burning charcoal is the same *gas silvestre*; but this was also

"a random conjecture. He does not even say that it ex-
"tinguishes flame; yet this was known to the chemists of
"his day. I had now the certain means of deciding the
"question, since, if the same, it must be fixed air. I made
"several indistinct experiments as soon as the conjecture
"occurred to my thoughts; but they were with little con-
"trivance or accuracy. In the evening of the same day that
"I discovered that it was fixed air that escaped from fer-
"menting liquors I made an experiment which satisfied me.
"Unfixing the muzzle of a pair of chamber bellows, I put a
"bit of charcoal, just red-hot, into the wide end of it, and then
"quickly putting it into its place again, I plunged the pipe
"to the bottom of a phial, and forced the air very slowly
"through the charcoal, so as to maintain its combustion, but
"not produce a heat too suddenly for the phial to bear. When
"I judged that the air of the phial was completely vitiated,
"I poured lime water into it, and had the pleasure of seeing it
"become milky in a moment.

   "I now admired van Helmont's sagacity, or his fortunate
"conjecture; and, for some years, I took it for granted that
"all those vapours which extinguish flame, and are de-
"structive of animal life, without irritating the lungs or giving
"warning by their converse nature are the *gas silvestre* of van
"Helmont or fixed air."

   It is thus evident that Black so early as 1757, the year
Haller published the first volume of his *Elementa*, had rediscovered the gas sylvestre of van Helmont, and to a certain
extent learned its nature. He recognized it as a distinct gas,
as something which, though it might be present in atmospheric air, was distinct from air, was not a mere modification
of air. He saw that it was irrespirable; and though he did not
lay hold of its nature with sufficient distinctness to justify
his calling it by the name applied to it much later and now
used by us, the name of carbonic acid gas, he proved by experiment that it arose from burning charcoal.

   Black recognized this fixed air as being present in ordinary
air, but he nowhere states to what extent it is so present. It
was, as we have seen, recognized by Mayow, by Haller, and
indeed generally that part only of the atmosphere was useful

for respiration. Mayow, as we have also seen, recognized this respirable part as distinct from the rest of the atmosphere; the others were not so clear, but in any case in the course of the century the words respirable air came into use. Black seems, and that very naturally, to have thought at first that the part of the atmosphere which was not respirable was his 'fixed air'; but he was led by a countryman of his to see that part of the atmosphere though not respirable was something quite different from his fixed air. He says in his *Treatise on Chemistry*:

"This portion of our atmosphere (the irrespirable portion, "that which the Swedish chemist, Scheele, had called foul air) "was first discovered in 1772 by my colleague Dr Rutherford "and published by him in his inaugural dissertation. He had "then discovered that we were mistaken in supposing that all "noxious air was the fixed air which I had discovered. He "says that after this has been removed by caustic alkali or "lime, a very large proportion of the air remains which ex- "tinguishes life and flame in an instant."

We may therefore say that *nitrogen* was discovered by Rutherford in 1772; but he did not give it this name, nor was he aware that this irrespirable constituent of the atmosphere had anything to do with the famous nitre which had so much occupied the minds of philosophers of the preceding century. It was not indeed until Cavendish, that eccentric nobleman, acute and careful observer, skilful experimenter, but strange being, obtained nitric acid from the atmosphere by electric sparking, that the connection between nitre and the chief constituent of the atmosphere became known. It was this connection which led the French chemist Chaptal to suggest for the atmospheric constituent the name nitrogen; but it was Lavoisier who first clearly defined its characters, and he always preferred to call it by a name which indicated its inability to sustain life, azotic gas or azote.

We have said that Black rediscovered under the title of fixed air the carbonic dioxide which van Helmont had dis- covered as gas sylvestre. We may similarly say that Priestley and Lavoisier rediscovered the gas which Mayow had made known by the name of igneo-aereal salt or spirit.

I need not here dwell at any length on the life of Joseph
Priestley. Born in 1733 at Fieldhead near Leeds, in York-
shire, educated to be a minister in the Unitarian Church, at
first a somewhat 'stickit' minister in Suffolk and in Cheshire,
afterwards holding a more congenial post as tutor in the
academy at Warrington, for some time literary companion
to Lord Shelburne, his most active life was spent as minister
first at Leeds, then at Birmingham. Man of letters as well
as man of science, prolific theologian and ardent politician,
his views did not commend themselves to the people, or shall
I rather say to the populace; as is well known he had to flee
from Birmingham, and after hiding somewhile in London
passed over to America and took up his abode at Northum-
berland in Pennsylvania, where in 1804 he died.

Priestley's first work on respiration consisted in attempts
to restore, to render once more respirable, air which had been
vitiated, rendered irrespirable by being breathed. After
several failures he at last succeeded by means of vegetation.
He says:

"I have been so happy as by accident to have hit upon a
"method of restoring air which has been injured by the
"burning of candles, and to have discovered at least one of
"the restoratives which nature employs for this purpose. It
"is *vegetation*.

*   *   *   *   *   *   *

"One might have imagined that, since common air is
"necessary to vegetable as well as to animal life, both plants
"and animals had affected it in the same manner, and I own
"I had that expectation, when I first put a sprig of mint into
"a glass jar, standing inverted in a vessel of water: but when
"it had continued growing there for some months, I found
"that the air would neither extinguish a candle, nor was it
"at all inconvenient to a mouse which I put into it. The
"plant was not affected any otherwise than was the necessary
"consequence of its confined situation.

*   *   *   *   *   *   *

"Finding that candles would burn very well in air in which
"plants had grown a long time, and having had some reason

"to think that there was something attending vegetation
"which restored air that had been injured by respiration, I
"thought it was possible that the same process might also
"restore the air which had been injured by the burning of
"candles.

"Accordingly, on the 17th of August 1771, I put a sprig of
"mint into a quantity of air, in which a wax candle had burnt
"out, and found that on the 27th of that same month another
"candle burned perfectly well in it. This experiment I repeated,
"without the least variation in the event, not less than eight
"or ten times in the remainder of the summer.

*   *   *   *   *   *   *

"This restoration of air, I found, depended on the *vegetating*
"*state* of the plant; for though I kept a great number of the
"fresh leaves of mint in a small quantity of air in which
"candles had burnt out, and changed them frequently, for
"a long space of time, I could perceive no melioration in the
"state of the air."

About the same time, following up an experiment of Hales,
he prepared what he called nitrous air or nitrous acid, and he
made the remarkable observation that this nitrous acid in
producing certain effects on air acted only on air fit for
respiration. He says:

"One of the most conspicuous properties of this kind of air
"is the great diminution of any quantity of common air with
"which it is mixed, attended with a turbid red, or deep
"orange colour and also a considerable heat.

*   *   *   *   *   *   *

"I hardly know any experiment that is more adapted to
"amaze and surprise than this is, which exhibits a quantity of
"air, which, as it were, devours a quantity of another kind of
"air, half as large as itself, and yet is so far from gaining any
"addition to its bulk, that it is considerably diminished by it."

He found this nitrous air could be conveniently used as
a test of the fitness of air for breathing. Either of these lines
of inquiry might have led him to the discovery which he
afterwards made. But they did not. His mind was too full of
phlogiston, and under the idea that common air consisted of

acid gas and phlogiston, he pursued long inquiries into other
acid gases than the nitrous air, into marine acid air, vitriolic
acid air, and even vegetable or acetous acid air.

These inquiries did not lead far; but another independent
inquiry suddenly brought him, accidentally as it were, upon
his great discovery.

He obtained after some difficulty an adequate burning-
glass such as would enable him to raise to the requisite heat
bodies enclosed in a glass vessel, the gases developed in which
he could study with success. By the help of this burning-
glass he, following up Hales' views, "tried to find out what
"kind of air a great variety of substances natural and artificial
"would yield."

While engaged on this inquiry, which was quite independent
of his earlier researches, he found that mercuric oxide, *mercurius calcinatus per se*, yielded under the action of the sun's
rays a quantity of gas which was not inflammable, and which
so far from quenching flame was exceedingly favourable for
combustion. These are his words:

"With this apparatus, after a variety of other experiments,
"an account of which will be found in its proper place, on the
"1st August, 1774, I endeavoured to extract air from *mer-
"curius calcinatus per se*; and I presently found that, by
"means of this lens, air was expelled from it very readily.
"Having got about three or four times as much as the bulk
"of my materials, I admitted water to it, and found that it
"was not imbibed by it. But what surprised me more than
"I can yet well express, was that a candle burned in this air
"with a remarkably vigorous flame, very much like that of
"the enlarged flame with which a candle burns in nitrous air,
"exposed to iron or liver of sulphur; but as I had got nothing
"like this remarkable appearance from any kind of air besides
"this particular modification of nitrous air, and I knew no
"nitrous acid was used in the preparation of *mercurius calci-
"natus*, I was utterly at a loss how to account for it."

He further mentions that "the flame of the candle, besides
"being larger, burned with more splendour and heat than in
"that species of nitrous air; and a piece of red-hot wood
"sparkled in it."

He obtained the same gas from red precipitate and from nimium; he found that a mouse lived well in it, and on trying it with his nitrous air he found that it was much better than, four or five times as good as, common air. It was therefore not common air, it was the same thing as that which renders common air fit for respiration, but as it were in a more condensed form.

Priestley, as I have said, was devoted to the phlogiston theory. He thought phlogiston; he could not lay hold of any subject save from the phlogiston point of view. Air supported combustion because it took up the phlogiston given out by the burning body. Common air was to a certain extent free from phlogiston, it was dephlogisticated, and in proportion as it was so dephlogisticated, it could support combustion. Common air supported combustion to a certain extent only, a part only of it could support combustion because it was only partially dephlogisticated. The new air which he got from the metallic oxides was wholly dephlogisticated.

"I got air," says he, "which I was gradually satisfied had "all the properties of common air, only in much greater "perfection, so as to be entitled (according to my idea of "purity or impurity with respect to air) to the name of "dephlogisticated air, which for that reason I gave to it."

He recognized the new thing which he had got not as a new thing, a new gas or air, different from the rest of the atmosphere, but as a part of the atmosphere brought into a new condition.

He thus in 1774 prepared oxygen, he prepared the igneo-aereal substance of Mayow, but he did not discover it, in the sense that he did not discover the true nature of the substance which he had prepared; what he did discover was that the air which he had prepared was that part of common air which supported combustion and life.

By the help of this discovery he could now explain on the phlogiston theory his previous results.

Animals whose bodies abound in phlogiston, introduced by their food (for both the dead food and the body which eats the food are combustible, and combustible means holding phlogiston), in the act of breathing give out phlogiston so long

as the atmosphere they breathe contains enough dephlogisticated air to absorb the phlogiston; when this dephlogisticated
air becomes saturated with phlogiston and can receive no
more, the atmosphere ceases to be respirable.

Animals can take in, can imbibe phlogiston only as part
of their food, can take it in only when it is already combined
with the substance of their food. Plants, on the other hand,
under the influence of light can imbibe phlogiston directly
from the air, can withdraw phlogiston from and so dephlo-
gisticate the air; hence it is that they can render respirable
or dephlogisticated the air which animals have rendered
irrespirable or phlogisticated. But they can do this only under
the influence of light.

"In these experiments," his experiments on air, "it clearly
"appeared that respiration is a *phlogistic process* affecting air
"in the very same manner as every other phlogistic process
"(viz. putrefaction, the effervescence of iron-filings and brim-
"stone, or the calcination of metals, etc.) affects it; diminishing
"the quantity of it in a certain proportion, lessening its
"specific gravity, and rendering it unfit for respiration or
"inflammation, but leaving it in a state capable of being
"restored to a tolerable degree of purity by agitation in
"water, etc."

The last words in the above sentence refer to some earlier
experiments made before he had observed the restoration of
vitiated air by vegetation, experiments which led him to
think that he could obtain a certain amount of restoration
by mere agitation with water.

He many times insists that respiration and putrefaction are
the same things.

"Respiration and putrefaction affect common air in the
"same manner, and in the same manner in which all noxious
"processes diminish air and make it noxious, and which agree
"in nothing but the emission of phlogiston. If this be the
"case it should seem that the phlogiston which we take in
"with our aliment, after having discharged its proper function
"in the animal system (by which it probably undergoes some
"unknown alteration) is discharged as effete by the lungs into
"the great common *menstruum*, the atmosphere."

He saw, moreover, in the changes of the colour of blood a confirmation of his views. Venous blood he took to be blood laden with phlogiston; this reaching the lungs parted with its phlogiston to the dephlogisticated part of the inspired air in the lungs, and went on its way as dephlogisticated blood to gather up phlogiston once more as it coursed through the body. A proof of this view he saw in the fact that blood exposed to dephlogisticated air gave up its phlogiston and became bright arterial dephlogisticated blood. Arterial blood exposed to phlogisticated air became phlogisticated, dark, and venous.

"Having taken the blood of a sheep...I introduced pieces "of the crassamentum, contained in nets of open gauze, "sometimes through water, and sometimes through quick- "silver, into different kinds of air, and always found that the "blackest part assumed a florid red colour in common air, "and more especially in dephlogisticated air, which is purer "and more fit for respiration than common air (and accord- "ingly the blood always acquired a more florid colour, and "the change was produced in less time in this than in common "air); whereas the brightest red blood became presently black "in any kind of air that was unfit for respiration, as in fixed "air, inflammable air, nitrous air or phlogisticated air; and "after having become black in the last of these kinds of air, "it regained its red colour upon being again exposed to "common air or to dephlogisticated air; the same pieces "becoming alternately black and red, by being transferred "from phlogisticated to dephlogisticated air; and *vice versâ*.

"In these experiments the blood must have parted with its "phlogiston to the common air or dephlogisticated air, and "have imbibed it and have become saturated with it when "exposed to phlogisticated, nitrous, inflammable, or fixed "air."

It will be observed that Priestley's idea of respiration as being simply the phlogistication of dephlogisticated air left no room for any other product of respiration. Black, we have seen, had clearly shewn that his fixed air was a product of respiration, was a constituent of expired air. Priestley (and this shews how far he was from laying hold of the real truth about respiration) had to explain away in some manner or other Black's fixed air. He attempts to shew that it does not come from the lungs.

"It now being pretty clearly determined that common air "is made to deposit the fixed air which entered into the "constitution of it by means of phlogiston in all cases of "diminished air, it will follow that in the precipitation of lime "by breathing into lime water the fixed air, which incor- "porates with lime, comes not from the lungs, but from the "common air, decomposed by the phlogiston exhaled from "them, and discharged, after having been taken in with the "aliment, and having performed its function in the animal "system."

Priestley's story is a striking example of the influence of a dominant theory. He was, as we have said, steeped in the phlogiston theory; he clung to it to the end of his life, though to others it seemed before that to have received its death-blow. From what I have said it is clear that he had formed in his mind an image of the respiratory process which, so far as oxygen is concerned, we with our present knowledge may call wonderfully exact, save that it was, in a sense, completely upside down, an image of the truth, but an inverted image. Where we say 'took,' he said 'give,' and *vice versâ*, and this so persistently throughout the whole business that anyone who attempts, as I have just done, to describe respiration in Priestley's terms, will find that he has to be very careful at each step lest he represent him as saying exactly the opposite of what he did say. It is so difficult for us, as it was so easy for him, to think of oxidation as a 'giving up,' and not as a 'taking in.'

Meanwhile another mind of quite a different mould was laying hold of the truth in its proper, erect position. Priestley was it is true a philosopher, a real investigator of nature, but he was also, and even more so, a politician and a theologian. In this latter side of his life the mode of thinking which he naturally adopted led him to regard every new fact which came before him as confirming the views at which he had already arrived, and perhaps especially encouraged him to expound the new fact as affording such welcome confirmation.

Possibly it was this other side of his mental activity which led him to cling so closely to the phlogiston faith. Indeed when we compare his character with that of Stahl, the founder of the phlogiston theory, we may see a certain likeness between the two.

The man who if he was not the first to prepare, was at least the first to discover oxygen, was free from all such tendencies to cling to old opinions. He was wholly and entirely the man of science holding to an old view only until the new one is ready, always prepared, at the bidding of a new indubitable fact, to throw aside at once his most cherished ideas.

I need not dwell long on the personal history, the private life of Antoine Laurent Lavoisier, and indeed there is little to tell save the tragic end of it.

Born on Aug. 26, 1743, he was educated at the Collège Mazarin. Here, though intended for the law, he was early drawn into studies of natural science; and to these he quietly devoted the rest of his life, spending his days, save those which he had to give up to official duties in connection with Le Ferme Général which he early took upon himself, in the researches of which I am about to speak, and in others which lie outside my present task. In 1768, at the early age of twenty-five, he was admitted into the Academy of Sciences, to which body he from time to time made known the brilliant results of his labours.

In 1775, the year after Priestley had prepared his dephlogisticated air, Lavoisier published the immortal paper 'On the nature of the principle which combines with metals during their calcination.' He saw the facts which Priestley had seen, but saw them eye to eye, saw them without the veil of preconceived ideas. The metallic oxide when it became a metal did not take up phlogiston from the air, but gave up something to the air. The metal when it was burnt into the oxide did not give up phlogiston to the air, it took something from the air. The metallic oxide in becoming metal, instead of gaining lost in weight. The metal in becoming metallic oxide, instead of losing gained in weight. Objections to the phlogiston theory based on questions of weight had been urged before, but the theory had swept them away. Now they were put in such a way that they swept away the theory. Smitten with these experiments the scientific Dagon, the image before which men had bowed their knees for a hundred years, fell crumbling to the ground.

Men will tell you tales of how Priestley, on a visit to Paris in the late autumn or winter of 1774, chatted freely to his scientific brethren about the experiment which he had just made with his mercuric oxide and his burning-glass; and they will assert that Lavoisier was thus led to his pregnant result. Whether this be true or no does not seem to me to be of vital importance; whether Lavoisier got at his result wholly of himself or no, he and he alone, not Priestley in any way, got at the true meaning of the result. He and he alone really discovered oxygen.

Two years later, in 1777, the year of Haller's death, in a paper entitled 'General Considerations concerning the Nature of Acids and on the Principles of which they are composed,' he brought forward abundant proofs that the principle which combines with metals when they are calcined, the dephlogisticated air of Priestley, is the constitutive principle of acidity.

"I shall therefore designate dephlogisticated air, air emi-"nently respirable, when in a state of combination or fixedness "by the name of 'acidifying principle,' or, if one prefers the "same meaning in a Greek dress, by that of 'oxygine' "principle."

In the same year, 1777, he attacked the problem of animal respiration in a paper, 'Experiments on the Respiration of Animals and on the Changes which the Air undergoes in passing through the lungs.'

Upon the discovery of oxygen and of the true nature of oxidation Priestley's image of the respiratory process forthwith inverted itself. It was seen at once that respiration was oxidation, that air which had been respired resembled air in which a metal had been calcined in so far that it had lost a certain quantity of its oxygen.

But Lavoisier went further than this, he saw that there was an essential difference between air in which a metal had been calcined and air which had been breathed. The latter contained what the former did not, Black's fixed air, for it precipitated lime water. Lavoisier, unlike Priestley, with no veil before his eyes, saw no reason to doubt that this fixed air came from the lungs; and he recognized accordingly that in respiration there were two factors, the disappearance of oxygen and the appearance of fixed air.

He took a measured quantity, 12 inches of vitiated air, of air which had been breathed, and passed it over caustic alkali. It was diminished in volume by $\frac{1}{6}$th, and the caustic alkali was found to have lost its causticity, and when treated with acid to give off fixed air. Lavoisier found that Black's fixed air could be most readily prepared by treating chalk with acids, and he had determined that it gave an acid reaction; hence he preferred to call it aeriform calcic acid. Hence he states the conclusion to be derived from the experiment just quoted in the following terms: "Air vitiated by breathing "contains $\frac{1}{6}$th part of an aeriform acid like that which is "obtained from chalk."

After this aeriform acid has been removed the air becomes exactly like the air in which a metal has been calcined, it is an air which extinguishes flame and is unfit for being breathed. This residual air, since it would not support life, Lavoisier proposed to call azotic air or azote. When this azote was mixed, to the extent of $\frac{1}{4}$th its volume, with air eminently respirable, dephlogisticated air (he did not as yet feel justified in using largely his new term oxygine), it became exactly like common air, the air of the atmosphere.

He draws from his experiments the following physiological conclusion:

"Either the portion of the air eminently respirable con-
"tained in the air of the atmosphere is converted into aeriform
"calcic acid, or a change is effected in the lung by which on
"the one hand the air eminently respirable is absorbed, and
"on the other hand the lung substitutes in its place in nearly
"equal volume a portion of aeriform calcic acid. I shewed
"during Easter 1775 that air eminently respirable could be
"entirely converted into aeriform calcic acid by the power of
"charcoal, and in other memoirs I shewed the same fact by
"other means" (that is to say, he had proved that Black's

fixed air was a compound of carbon and oxygen). "This makes "the former of the two views possible. On the other hand it "is also possible that the air eminently respirable combines "with the blood. We know that it is a property of the air "eminently respirable to communicate a red colour to the "bodies with which it combines, especially metallic substances, "as, for example, mercury, lead, and iron. May we not con-"clude that the red colour of blood is due to a combination "of the air eminently respirable, or more exactly, as I shall "shew in a memoir shortly to appear, to the combination of "the base of the air eminently respirable with an animal "liquid, in the same way that the red colour of red mercury "precipitate and nimium is due to a combination of the base "of the same air with a metallic substance? For Priestley "has shewn that blood becomes red when exposed to air "eminently respirable, and dark when exposed to aeriform "calcic acid; in the latter case becoming red again when "exposed once more to air eminently respirable.

"We may therefore regard as proved,

"1. Respiration affects only the air eminently respirable; "the rest of the atmosphere, the mephitic part," the part which he later called azote, "remains unchanged.

"2. The calcination of metals in atmospheric air goes on "until the air eminently respirable contained in the atmo-"sphere is exhausted and combined with the metal, but will "not go on afterwards.

"3. Animals shut up in a confined atmosphere succumb, "so soon as they have absorbed or converted into aeriform "calcic acid the greater part of the respirable portion of the "atmosphere, leaving a remainder.

"4. This remainder is the same in calcination and in respi-"ration, provided that in the latter case the aeriform calcic "acid be removed; and in any case is reconverted into "ordinary atmospheric air by adding to it air eminently "respirable.

"If we augment or diminish in any atmosphere the quantity "of air eminently respirable, we augment or diminish the "quantity of metal which can be calcined in it, and to a cer-"tain extent the time during which the animal can live in it."

Thus at a single stroke as it were did this clear-sighted inquirer solve the problem of oxidation, and almost, if not quite, the problem of respiration. He brought our knowledge of the latter process very nearly to its present condition.

Yet he went still a step further.

Three years later, in 1780, he and the great mathematician Laplace published their celebrated memoir on heat.

In this memoir these authors, after placing the theory of the heat of oxidation and combustion on a sound basis, after describing their methods for determining the heat given out during chemical action, the results which they obtained, and the conclusions to be derived from those results, applied their new views to elucidate the cause of the natural heat of living bodies.

As we have seen, Haller left the problem of animal heat in an unsettled condition. The chemical theories of its origin had fallen somewhat into disrepute; but the mechanical theory, that it was due to the friction of the blood in its movements, though favoured by Haller did not seem to him to be wholly satisfactory.

Black, besides discovering fixed air, had prepared the way for the true theory of heat by pointing out the distinction between latent and sensible heat, and had introduced the ideas of capacity for heat and of specific heat. In 1777–9 Adair Crawford published a theory of heat, based on Black's views; a theory which, as he put it forward, seems vague and hypothetical, but which at least has the merit of connecting animal heat and respiration in a way which had not been done before. His theory was as follows:

Inspired air contains elementary fire, and meets in the lungs with the inflammable principle present in the blood. The elementary fire leaves the air of the lungs to join the blood, the capacity for heat of which is increased. In the course of the circulation the blood again becomes impregnated with the inflammable principle by which the capacity of the blood for heat is diminished. It accordingly gives up heat to the tissues. Thus in the lungs the blood discharges inflammable principle and absorbs heat, in the system it imbibes this principle and emits heat.

It must be remembered that Black and Crawford, and indeed Lavoisier, regarded heat or caloric not, as we now do, as a form of energy, but as a thing or substance which com- bined with the thing heated, a something which was the physical analogue of the chemical phlogiston.

Very different from Crawford's loose hypothesis is Lavoisier's clear and succinct statement of the results of his and Laplace's experiments. Having ascertained the amount of heat given out by the combustion of a given weight of carbon into what now began to be called not aeriform calcic acid but carbonic acid gas, so quickly did knowledge advance in these few pregnant years, and having determined on the one hand how much carbonic acid was given out by, that is to say how much carbon underwent combustion in the body of an animal during a given time, and on the other hand how much heat was given out by the animal during the same time, the authors found on comparing the results, that the heat given out by the animal was about the same as that given out by a quantity of carbon oxidized so as to produce the amount of carbonic acid gas expired by the animal during the time.

They thus felt justified in stating the following conclusion. "Respiration is therefore a combustion, slow it is true, but "otherwise perfectly similar to the combustion of charcoal. "It takes place in the interior of the lung without giving rise "to sensible light because the matter of the fire (the caloric), "as soon as it is set free, is forthwith absorbed by the humidity "of these organs. The heat developed by this combustion is "communicated to the blood which is traversing the lungs, "and from the lungs is distributed over the whole animal "system."

A few years later, in 1785, Lavoisier was led to recognize that he had been in error in supposing that respiration was a combustion of carbon only. In a memoir entitled 'The Changes undergone by Respired Air,' he made a careful quantitative estimation of the quantity of oxygen (or 'vital air,' as he still preferred to call it, being unlike some other makers of new terms chary of using his new word, oxygine) which disappeared when an animal was made to breathe a

measured atmosphere of it for a given time. He also esti-
mated the quantity of carbonic acid gas given out during the
same time; and knowing by this time the exact composition
of carbonic acid, knowing how much oxygen was present in
a given quantity of carbonic acid, he found that all the oxygen
which disappeared did not reappear in the carbonic acid respired. Some of the oxygen was used for something else than
the combustion of carbon and the production of carbonic acid.

Now in expired air there was nothing present in measurable
quantity except carbonic acid and the substance known as
water.

Here I must go back a little.

Van Helmont found that his gas, of which, as seen in gas
sylvestre, the conspicuous feature was that it would not
support burning, though sometimes uninflammable, sometimes caught fire and burnt. Boyle in 1672 recognized that
the air or gas given off when metals were dissolved in acids
was inflammable. And during the eighteenth century mention
is from time to time made of factitious air, and of this air
being often inflammable. Hales refers to it; and Haller speaks
of factitious air, such as is produced by the action of acids
on metals, and is frequently inflammable, as being unfit for
respiration, although it is elastic. As we have seen, Haller
attributed much importance in respiration to the fact that air
in being breathed lost its elastic power, and thought the
possession of elastic power a feature of respirable air; hence he
found a difficulty in elastic factitious air not being respirable.

It is with Cavendish however, and his experiments on
factitious air in 1766, that our real, exact knowledge of inflammable factitious air begins; and when in 1781 he discovered the composition of water, this mysterious gas became
henceforth known as *hydrogen*. It was the last of the four
chief physiological gases to be run to earth. As we have seen,
carbonic acid gas first laid hold of van Helmont in 1640 or
thereabouts, was more firmly grasped by Black in 1757.
Nitrogen was first observed by Rutherford in 1772. Oxygen,
prepared by Priestley in 1774, was recognized by Lavoisier
in 1775, and hydrogen was first made definite and clear by
Cavendish in 1781.

Thus in 1785 hydrogen was well known to Lavoisier, and he was able to draw from the quantitative comparison of which I have just been speaking the following important conclusion:
"Besides the part converted into carbonic acid a portion "of the inspired vital air does not issue as it enters. There "results therefore one of two things; this part either unites "with the blood or combines (in the lungs) with a portion of "hydrogen to form water."

Had Lavoisier stopped here we should have been able to say not only that he had in a most masterly manner solved the general problem of respiration, but that every jot and tittle of his work remained true and good for all time since his day. He was however a little later on led into a false path. In 1790 he published in conjunction with the physiologist Sequin a memoir on 'The Transpiration of Animals.' In that memoir the authors give a luminous though brief exposition of the new views which had been reached of the chemistry of the body. They explain how digestion supplies the blood with the material for combustion, with carbon and hydrogen, how that material undergoes combustion, is oxidized by the respiratory process, thus giving forth heat, and how the products of that combustion, water and carbonic acid, are got rid of through the skin and lungs. They clearly recognize that part only of the water thus thrown off comes from the oxidation of hydrogen, indeed a small part only, the rest being merely the water which serves as the vehicle of the solid food. The exposition is quite a modern one save in one point. In the discussion on the oxidation of respiration there occurs this remarkable sentence, "one must know in "the first place that there transudes into the bronchi a "humour which is secreted from the blood and which is "principally composed of carbon and hydrogen."

The view put forward is that the oxidation of the carbon and hydrogen supplied by the food takes place within the lungs, in the tubes of the lungs, as the oxidation of a hydro-carbonous fluid secreted into the tubes.

Now Lavoisier was no anatomist, was not indeed a physiologist, and in his other writings does not venture into physiological as distinct from chemical hypotheses. One cannot help suspecting that he was led astray into this wrong hypothesis by his more distinctly physiological comrade. However it be, the idea of the hydrocarbonous fluid laid hold of men's minds, and was accepted as an integral part of the new doctrine of respiration: accepted, but not by all. In the following year, 1791, Hassenfratz, a chemist of some reputation, who had been assistant to Lavoisier, and was now assistant to the mathematician Lagrange, in a paper in the *Annales de Chimie*, 'On the combination of oxygen with the carbon and the hydrogen of the blood; on the solution of the oxygen in the blood; and on the manner in which caloric is set free,' expounds the following view of respiration as put forward by Lagrange: "M. Lagrange reflecting that if all the "heat which is distributed in the animal economy was set free "in the lungs, the temperature of the lungs would therefore "necessarily be raised so much that one would have reason "to fear they would be destroyed, and that moreover were "the temperature of the lungs so much higher than that of "other parts, this fact could hardly have escaped observation, "concluded accordingly with great probability that the heat "of the animal economy was set free not in the lungs alone, "but in all parts of the body where the blood circulated."

Lagrange supposed therefore that the blood in passing through the lungs dissolved the oxygen of the inspired air, and that this dissolved oxygen was carried away by the blood into the arteries and thence into the veins, and that "in the "course of the journey of the blood the oxygen little by little "quitted the condition of solution in order to combine in part "with the carbon and in part with the hydrogen of the blood, "and so to form carbonic acid and water, which are set free "from the venous blood so soon as this leaves the right side "of the heart to enter the lungs." And Hassenfratz relates, in support of Lagrange's view, experiments of his own, on the changes in colour of blood when exposed to oxygen on the one hand, and to carbonic acid on the other; but these, which are in the main repetitions of Priestley's earlier experiments, do not amount to much.

It will be observed that Lagrange's view is the modern view, except that we have since learnt that the oxidation takes place, not in the blood itself, but in the elements of the tissue outside the blood channels. Yet this view was not accepted by all, or even generally, for some time. For many years Lavoisier's view, or rather Sequin's, held its ground. Even the hypothetical hydrocarbonous fluid was accepted, though some, while still maintaining that the oxidation took place in the lungs, supposed that the carbon and hydrogen were oxidised while still in the blood of the pulmonary vessels, and did not need any preliminary secretion into the pulmonary passages.

The acute Spallanzani, laying hold of Lavoisier's discoveries so soon as they were made known, devoted much time during the latter years of his life to numerous experiments on the respiration of animals, both vertebrate and invertebrate; the memoirs embodying the results which he had obtained were not published however until after his death, namely in 1803. In addition to many valuable observations as to the effects of circumstances and environment, such as temperature, hybernation and the like on the respiratory process, these memoirs contain two far-reaching conclusions. The one is that the tissues, like the body as a whole, respire, that is to say consume oxygen and produce carbonic acid; the other is that animals (snails) placed in an atmosphere of hydrogen or nitrogen give out carbonic acid in the same way that they do in common air.

These results really overthrew Lavoisier's theory of a hydrocarbonous secretion; but they failed to produce their proper effect, even when put forward in a more complete form many years later, in 1823, by W. F. Edwards, in his striking essay, 'The influence of physical agents on life.' The view that oxidation took place in the lungs, and not in the body generally, continued to hold its own, mainly for the reason that, owing to imperfect experimental methods, the various attempts made to shew that blood, as demanded by Lagrange's theory, contained on the one hand oxygen and on the other hand carbonic acid gas, fell short of decisive results. It was not until 1837 when Gustav Magnus, making use of the mercurial air-pump, definitely proved that both venous and arterial blood contained both these gases, though in different proportions, that the theory of respiration assumed the form in which we now hold it.

Lavoisier made no reply to Lagrange; and there were reasons why he did not.

While quite a young man, he had, against the advice of many of his scientific friends, become connected with the Ferme Général, as adjoint to the Fermier Baudon; and in the midst of his glorious scientific activity he had developed remarkable administrative powers. He did notable work of this kind in connection with the Government manufacture of gunpowder. His last memoir on matters connected with respiration, the one just mentioned as written with Sequin, was read before the Academy of Sciences in April 1790. This and other of his work had been done in the midst of the earlier storm and whirlwind of the Revolution.

The storm was now thickening, the whirlwind was growing wilder, the days of the great terror were coming on, and Lavoisier, and indeed the Academy, began to have enemies among the sons of the people. In 1792 Fourcroy proposed to purge the Academy of those suspected of leanings towards the old order of things. In 1793, the Convention suppressed it. In those dark days Lavoisier laboured hard to help others in the work of science, but in the tumult he found no opportunity for quiet research. And soon all opportunity was to be taken away from him for ever.

The Convention arrested Lavoisier and his colleagues, and on May 8, 1794, these were put on their trial and condemned. Execution was swift. On the morning of May the 9th there passed in carts from the Conciergerie to the Place de la Révolution a procession of men to meet their death. As the sharp stroke of the guillotine severed in turn the neck of the fourth of these, there passed away from this world, in his fifty-first year, this master-mind of science, who had done so much to draw aside from truth the veil of man's ignorance and wrong thought, and there passed away too the hope of his drawing aside yet other folds of that veil, folds which perhaps wrap us round even to-day.

LECTURE X

THE OLDER DOCTRINES OF THE
NERVOUS SYSTEM

I NOW wish to turn to the views which have been held in
the past concerning the brain and the rest of the nervous
system, and concerning the way in which by means of it
sensation and movement are carried out. I cannot do better
than start with the views which were held by Vesalius.

Vesalius expounds his views on the nervous system as
follows:

"As therefore the power of the vital soul (that is the sum
"total of the vital spirit, or the vital spirit regarded as a
"whole) is situated in the substance of the heart, and the
"power of the natural soul in the proper substance of the
"liver, and as the liver prepares the cruder blood together
"with the natural spirit, and the heart the purer blood, which
"together with the vital spirit rushes with speed throughout
"the body, and as these viscera by means of the canals
"allotted to them distribute their products to all parts of the
"body, so also does the brain in appropriate structures, and
"in organs properly subserving its work, manufacture the
"animal spirit which is by far the brightest and most delicate,
"and indeed is a quality rather than an actual thing. And
"while on the one hand it employs this spirit for the opera-
"tions of the chief soul, on the other hand it is continually
"distributing it to the instruments of the senses and of move-
"ment by means of nerves, as it were by cords, the soul never
"being lacking in this spirit which may be regarded as the
"chief author of the activity of those instruments, any more
"certainly than the liver and heart ever leave wholly destitute,
"at least in health, any of the parts on which they bestow
"their products, although they do not always supply them
"either in the same quantity or the same quality. Nerves
"therefore serve the same purpose to the brain that the great
"artery does to the heart, and the vena cava to the liver, in as
"much as they convey to the instruments to which it ought
"to be sent the spirit prepared by the brain, and hence may be
"regarded as the busy attendants and messengers of the brain.

"The material, however, for the animal spirit is supplied
"by the vital spirit, abounding as this does in the arteries
"which in numerous series reach both the hard and the thin
"membrane (dura mater and arachnoid) investing the brain,
"as also by the air which in breathing is drawn in towards
"the brain, on the one hand through the minute holes drilled
"in the sixth (or ethmoid) bone of the skull for the special
"purpose of smell, and on the other hand through those
"orifices in the skull which look towards the palate, as we
"explained very early in this work. And indeed air where
"it can find an entrance makes its way into the right and left
"ventricles of the brain, and into the one which lies between
"these. This vital spirit, although we may regard it as being
"very abundant in all the vessels and sinuses of the mem-
"branes of the brain is however chiefly brought into the right
"and left ventricles of the brain by the larger branches of the
"arteries which are directed to the sides of the gland receiving
"the mucus of the brain (the pituitary gland); offsets from
"these imbedded in processes of the thin membrane enter
"the lower parts of the right and left ventricle and then make
"their way over their whole extent. But besides these
"arteries a particular vessel from the fourth sinus of the
"membrana dura, passing under the body which resembles
"in shape a turtle or a chamber built in the form of an arch,
"reaches the front part of the brain by the cavity which is
"common to the right and left ventricles. This after several
"flexures divides at length into two parts, one of which passes
"to the right and the other to the left ventricle, and so joins
"the arteries of that situation, forming a net which resembles
"the membranes of the foetus more than anything else.

"From the air which has thus made its way into the brain,
"and from the vital spirit which on account of the numerous
"flexures becomes more and more fitted for the use of the
"brain, the animal spirit is by the special power of the brain
"elaborated in the right and left ventricles, and in the cavity
"common to the two known as the third ventricle. A portion
"(of this animal spirit) is carried from this third ventricle,
"directed through the oblong channel (aqueduct of Sylvius)
"between the bodies which resemble the nates and testes to

"the ventricle of the cerebellum (fourth ventricle) which is
"formed by the sinus of the cerebellum, and partly by the
"cavity of the beginning of the dorsal medulla (spinal cord).
  "From this ventricle no mean portion of the animal spirit
"is directed into the dorsal medulla and into the nerves
"springing from it. From the other ventricles of the brain
"however the spirit is carried into the nerves springing directly
"from them, and so to the organs of the senses and voluntary
"movement.
  "Meanwhile, we will not too anxiously discuss whether the
"spirit is carried along certain hollow channels of the nerves,
"as the vital spirit is carried by the arteries, or whether it
"passes through the solid material of the nerves, as light passes
"through the air. But in any case it is through the nerves
"that the influence of the brain is brought to bear on any part,
"so far I can certainly follow out the functions of the brain
"by means of vivisections, with great probability and indeed
"truth."
  In his chapter on vivisections, he shews how by cutting or
ligaturing this or that nerve you can abolish the action of this
or that muscle, or how having ligatured a number of nerves,
by loosing now this and now that ligature, you can bring this
and that muscle into action again, all shewing that the contraction of the muscle is dependent on its nerve. He mentions
incidentally that you may divide a muscle lengthwise without
stopping its contraction, but if you cut it crosswise, you do
interfere in proportion to the depth of the cut. He shews that
it is the nerve itself which is the essential agent, and not its
membranes, for you may remove the membranes without
interfering with movement. He further shews that if you lay
bare the dorsal medulla (spinal cord), and cut it across, all
the parts supplied with nerves leaving the medulla below the
section will be deprived of sensation and movement.
  In the chapter on the brain from which we were quoting
he continues thus:
  "But how the brain performs its functions in imagination,
"in reasoning, in thinking and in memory (or in whatever
"way, following the dogmas of this or that man, you prefer
"to classify or name the several actions of the chief soul), I

"can form no opinion whatever. Nor do I think that any-
"thing more will be found out by anatomy or by the methods
"of those theologians who deny to brute animals all power
"of reasoning, and indeed all the faculties belonging to what
"we call the chief soul. For as regards the structure of the
"brain, the monkey, dog, horse, cat, and all quadrupeds
"which I have hitherto examined, and indeed all birds, and
"many kinds of fish, resemble man in almost every particular.
"Nor do we by dissection come upon any difference which
"would indicate that the functions of those animals should
"be treated otherwise than those of man; unless perchance
'anyone says, and that rightly, that the mass of the brain
"attains its highest dimensions in man, which we know to be
"the most perfect animal, and that his brain is found to be
"bigger than that of three oxen; and then in proportion to
"the size of the body, first the ape, and next the dog exhibit
"a large brain, suggesting that animals excel in the size of
"their brains in proportion as they seem the more openly and
"clearly to be endowed with the faculties of the chief soul.
"Indeed the more I examine the nature of the heart, the liver,
"the testes, and the organs secondary to these, the functions
"performed by which are, there can be no doubt, the same
"in us as in other animals, and the more I persuade myself
"that we ought not to draw conclusions concerning the opera-
"tions of the chief soul, other than those taught by our most
"holy and true religion, the more I wonder at what I read
"in the scholastic theologians and the lay philosophers con-
"cerning the three ventricles with which they say the brain
"is supplied."

And then he goes on to ridicule the view held by these
philosophers, namely that a front ventricle is the receptacle
of sensations which, passed on to a second ventricle in the
middle of the head, are there used for imagination, reasoning
and thought, and that a third ventricle near the back of the
head is devoted to memory. "Of such a kind are the figments
"of men who have never studied the handiwork of God the
"maker of all things as seen in the structure of bodies, but
"who take to themselves reckless opinions gathered from all
"manner of sources, figments imagined surely not without

"grave impiety. How wrong these are in their description "of the structure of the brain the following discourse will "shew."

It is obvious that Vesalius took a distinctly physiological view of the origin of the chief soul. The chief soul is to him the totality of the animal spirits just as the vital soul is the totality of the vital spirits; it is engendered in the brain by "virtue of the powers of the proper material and form of the "brain," just as the vital soul is engendered by the substance of the heart; or as we should say in modern language, psychical phenomena are the outcome of the activity of the nervous tissues. And from the way in which he not once only but repeatedly scoffs at the philosophers who deny to brute beasts all the principal functions of the chief soul, though the brains of these are so like that of man, we may infer that he nursed in secret the belief that future inquiry would make clear the hidden meaning of the complicated structure of the brain, and shew how its several parts were concerned in the different activities of the soul. But the time for that had not yet come. Even the preliminary step, an adequate psychological analysis of the faculties of the soul, was as in his opinion yet wanting; and he refused to waste his time in speculations, the conclusions of which could not be tested either by anatomical observation or by vivisectional experiment. He was clear that the soul was engendered in and by the brain, but beyond that he knew next to nothing. Vivisection taught him that when the brain is removed, sensation and movement are lost; but it taught him little more than this. He was not to be led into a quarrel with the Church, by indulging in speculations having no solid basis. "And so the learned anatomist trained "in the dissection of dead bodies, and tainted with no heresy, "will readily understand how little I should be consulting "my own interests were I to lecture on the results to be "obtained by the vivisection of the brain, which otherwise "I would most willingly have done, and indeed at great "length."

In this as in almost everything else which Vesalius wrote there is a wholly modern ring. We seem to be stepping backwards again when nearly a hundred years later we come to the views of van Helmont and Descartes. I put these together, for the sensitive and motive soul of van Helmont and the rational soul of Descartes, though the latter includes van Helmont's immortal mind, are alike in this that they are both outside and distinct from the animal spirits, the activities of the nervous tissues themselves. That the seat of the soul is placed by one in the pylorus and by the other in the pineal gland is a matter of indifference. The essential point of both views is that the soul is something added to, different from the mere results of the action of the tissues of the brain. This permitted Descartes to accept and make use of the strictest physical conceptions of the nervous phenomena themselves.

To Descartes the whole body was nothing but a machine whose motive power lay in that heat which was innate in the heart though fed and sustained by the food carried to it in the blood; in this respect he, rejecting the modern doctrines of Harvey and others, followed the teaching of the ancients. To him the whole body was nothing but a machine, in which the blood, heated and rarefied in the heart, engendered "the "very subtle air or rather the very lively and pure flame, called "the animal spirits," which in turn in that part of the machine called the brain and nervous system on the one hand carried out according to simple physical and mechanical laws all the movements of the body in response to changes in the environment, and on the other hand, by supplying the physical basis for and by working on the rational soul, gave rise to modifications of thought.

Though he speaks of the animal spirits as an 'air' or a 'wind' or a 'flame,' yet throughout he treats them as if they constituted a fluid, a fluid very subtle indeed and of a wholly peculiar nature, but still a fluid and so far amenable to the physical laws governing fluids. It was in his time a doctrine daily gaining ground that the nerves were tubes along which the animal spirits flowed. Laying hold of this doctrine and making use of some known general facts of the topography of the brain and nerves, he constructs an ideal nervous machine consisting of the brain as a centre and of nervous tubes radiating from this centre and carrying the animal spirits to all parts of the body. And, in order to make the exposition of the working of this machine clear and convincing, he does not hesitate to attribute to its various parts features which he describes as if they belonged to the common knowledge of the time, though neither he nor anyone else had actually seen them.

His exposition of the general working of the machine is as follows:

"For you must know that the arteries which bring the "blood from the heart after having divided into an infinite "number of small branches and having formed the delicate "tissue which is spread like a carpet over the floor of the "ventricles of the brain, are gathered together round a certain "little *gland* which is placed about the middle of the sub- "stance of the brain, just at the entrance into the ventricles. "And these arteries have in this situation a large number of "minute orifices through which the more subtle particles of "the blood which they hold can flow into this gland but "which are so narrow that they do not permit any passage "through them of the grosser particles.

"You must also know that these arteries do not end there "but, being gathered together again, several into one, they "ascend straight upwards and join the great vessel, which "is like a Euripus, and which bathes the outer surface of the "brain. And it must be noticed that the grosser particles of "the blood lose a great deal of their agitation in the turns "and twists of the delicate tissue through which they pass, "the more so that they have the power to impinge on the "smaller more subtle particles mixed with them and to "transfer their movement to these. But these more delicate "particles are not able in the same way to lose their move- "ment, which indeed is increased by the movement trans- "ferred to them from the grosser particles, since there are "no other bodies in their neighbourhood to which the latter "can so easily transfer their movement.

"Hence it will be easily understood that these grosser "particles, as they ascend straight up towards the outer "surface of the brain where they serve for the nutrition of its "substance, bring it about that the more delicate and more "agitated particles are turned aside, and all enter into this

"gland, which must be regarded as a very full reservoir
"whence the spirits at the same time flow into the ventricles
"of the brain. Thus, without any other preparation or change
"except that they are separated from the grosser particles
"and that they still retain the extreme velocity which the
"heat of the heart has given them, they cease to have the
"form of blood and are called animal spirits.

   "Now as these spirits enter thus into the ventricles of the
"brain, so they pass thence into the pores of its substance and
"from these pores into the nerves. And according as they
"enter or even only as they tend to enter more or less into
"this or that nerve they have the power of changing the form
"of the muscle into which the nerve is inserted and by this
"means of making the limbs move. You may have seen in
"the grottoes and fountains which are in our royal gardens
"that the simple force with which the water moves in issuing
"from its source is sufficient to put into motion various
"machines and even to set various instruments playing or
"to make them pronounce words according to the varied
"disposition of the tubes which convey the water.

   "And indeed one may very well compare the nerves of the
"machine which I am describing with the tubes of the
"machines of these fountains, the muscles and tendons of the
"machine with the other various engines and springs which
"serve to move these machines, and the animal spirits, the
"source of which is the heart and of which the ventricles of
"the brain are the reservoirs, with the water which puts them
"in motion. Moreover breathing and other like acts which
"are natural and usual to the machine and which depend
"on the flow of the spirits are like the movements of a clock
"or of a mill which the ordinary flow of water can keep going
"continually. External objects, which by their mere presence
"act upon the organs of sense of the machine and which by
"this means determine it to move in several different ways
"according as the parts of the machine's brain are disposed,
"may be compared to strangers, who entering into one of the
"grottoes containing many fountains, themselves cause,
"without knowing it, the movements which they witness.
"For in entering they necessarily tread on certain tiles or

"plates, which are so disposed that if they approach a bathing
"Diana, they cause her to hide in the rose-bushes, and if they
"try to follow her, they cause a Neptune to come forward
"to meet them threatening them with his trident. Or if they
"pass in another direction they occasion the springing forward
"of a marine monster who spouts water into their faces, or
"things of a like kind according to the caprice of the engineers
"who constructed them.

"Lastly, when the rational soul resides in this machine, it
"has its principal seat in the brain and may be compared to
"the fountaineer who has to take his place in the reservoir
"whence all the various tubes of these machines proceed
"whenever he wishes to set them going, to stop them or in
"any way to change them."

Thus the pineal gland, "the little gland in the middle of
"the substance of the brain," is the primary reservoir, and the
ventricles of the brain form a secondary reservoir of the animal
spirits, which flowing from the brain along the tubular nerves
carry out the movements of the body, the energy of these
spirits being supplied by the innate heat of the heart. He
explains in the following manner the particular way in which
the working of this nervous machine is determined by the
impressions of external objects. The nerves are not mere
hollow tubes, provided with valvular arrangements by means
of which the flow of the animal spirits outwards from the
brain to the muscles and other structures is regulated; they
contain also within their cavities, delicate threads, forming
a sort of marrow, and these threads by centripetal action
determine the outflow of the spirits from the gland and from
the ventricles into the nerves.

"You see also that in each of these little tubes there is a
"sort of marrow composed of a large number of exceedingly
"delicate threads starting from the proper substance of the
"brain." (He explains elsewhere that the proper substance
of the brain forming the walls of the ventricles is composed of
an intricate network of these delicate threads, the meshes of
the network being the pores or mouths of the tubular nerves.)
"The ends of these threads terminate on the one hand at the
"internal surface of the brain looking towards the ventricles,

"and on the other hand in the skin or other tissues in which
"the tubes which hold them end. But, since this marrow does
"not serve for the movement of the members" (is not motor
in function as we should say but sensitive only), "it will be
"enough at the present moment if you know that it does not
"wholly fill the tube which holds it so that the animal spirits
"have ample room to flow readily from the brain to the muscles
"to which these little tubes, which ought here to be considered
"as so many little nerves, are distributed.

*   *   *   *   *

"Know then that a very large number of little threads like
"the above begin to separate all of them, the one from the
"other, at the internal surface of the brain where they take
"their origin, and spreading thence over all the rest of the
"body serve as organs of sense.

*   *   *   *   *

"In order to understand how the brain can be excited by
"external objects which affect the organs of sense, so that all
"the members can be moved in a thousand different ways,
"imagine that the delicate threads, which as I have already
"said arise from the inside of the brain and form the marrow
"of the nerves, are so disposed in all those parts which serve
"as the organs of any sense that they can easily be set in
"motion by the objects of the senses, and that, whenever
"they are thus set in motion, even ever so little, they, at the
"same instant, pull upon the parts of the brain whence they
"take origin, and by this means open up the orifices of certain
"pores which exist on the internal surface of the brain.
"Through these pores the animal spirits which are in the
"ventricles immediately begin to make their way and thus
"pass into the nerves and so into the muscles which carry
"out in the machine of which we are speaking movements
"exactly like those to which we ourselves are incited when our
"senses are affected in the same way.

"If for example fire comes near the foot, the minute
"particles of this fire which as you know move with great
"velocity, have the power to set in motion the spot of the
"skin of the foot which they touch, and by this means pulling

"upon the delicate thread which is attached to the spot of
"the skin, they open up at the same instant the pore against
"which the delicate thread ends, just as by pulling at one
"end of a rope one makes to strike at the same instant a bell
"which hangs on the other end."

According to Descartes then the movements of the body
viewed as 'an earthly machine' are brought about by that
part of the brain which forms the walls of ventricles serving
as centre where the play of sensitive impulses communicated
by the delicate threads of the marrow of the nerves determines the outflow of the motor animal spirits along the
tubular channels of the nerves. And making use of the
physical properties of the delicate threads on the one hand,
and of the subtle but powerful fluid, the animal spirits, on
the other hand, by the help by various devices such as
valvular arrangements in the nerves, the existence of which
he takes for granted, he gives a detailed exposition of the
varied working of the machine. He does not hesitate to
assume the existence in the nerves of various physical properties and to explain by means of them various nervous and
even psychical phenomena. He finds for instance the physical
basis for habit and memory in the following:

"Consider also that an important feature of these delicate
"threads is the property of being easily bent in every kind of
"way by the mere force of the spirits which press upon them
"and of retaining, just as if they were made of lead or of wax
"as it were, the shape into which they were last thrown until,
"by some further action, they are made to assume a new one."

The ventricles of the brain however do not form the only
reservoir of the animal spirits; another and more important
reservoir is the pineal gland. This moreover is the only part
of the brain to which is attached the rational soul; this is
"the seat of imagination and of common sensation." Through
it the rational soul can directly bring about body movements
and through it external objects are able to impress the soul.
He develops a mechanical theory explaining how the movements of the spirits from the surface of the pineal gland are
correlated to the movements of the spirits at the internal
surface of the ventricles, the entrance into the pores of the

latter affecting the outflow from the pores of the former, and
gives an interesting exposition of how in the action of external
objects on the delicate threads of the nerves there is a double
event, a primary event by which impulses from external
objects "impress their figure" on the internal surface of the
ventricles, and a secondary event by which a corresponding
figure is impressed on the surface of the pineal gland and so
on the soul. The first, serving as a relay, is as we should say
a purely nervous, the latter a psychical, event.

"Not those figures which are impressed on the external
"organs of the senses or on the inner surface of the ventricles
"of the brain, but only those which are traced in the spirits
"on the surface of the pineal gland can be considered as
"ideas, that is to say as the forms or images of which the
"rational soul will take direct cognizance, when, being
"united to the machine, it imagines or feels any object."

And he takes advantage of the mobility of the pineal gland
to offer a mechanical explanation of psychical phenomena.
"Consider moreover that the gland is composed of very soft
"material and that it is not completely joined and united to
"the substance of the brain but only attached to the small
"arteries (the walls of which are very loose and flexible) and
"that it is kept balanced by the force of the blood which the
"heat of the heart drives towards it. Hence it needs very
"little to determine it to incline or to lean now on this side,
"now on that, and to bring it about that in leaning it dis-
"poses the spirits which issue from it to direct themselves
"towards certain parts of the brain rather than towards
"others." The rush of spirits determined by the action of
the impression of an external object makes the pineal gland
lean on one side, the result of which is that, the disposition
of its pores being changed, these on the one hand permit a
freer outflow of certain spirits "so that the idea which these
"spirits form becomes more perfect," and on the other hand
hinder the issue of other spirits, moved by some other object
"so that you see, how one idea prevents another being
"received."

In anticipation as it were he rejects beforehand the views
which were later on brought forward by Stahl. Putting aside

the direct actions of the rational soul, all other vital phenomena are the results of pure machinery; he admits no necessity
to call in the aid of spiritual agencies to explain these; they
are to be explained like all other physical phenomena of the
universe, by the aid of the new mechanical philosophy.

This is what he says:

"All the functions of the body follow naturally from the
"sole disposition of its organs just in the same way that the
"movements of a clock or other self-acting machine, or auto-
"maton, follow from the arrangement of its weights and
"wheels. So that there is no reason on account of its functions
"to conceive that there exists in the body any soul whether
"vegetative or sensitive, or any principle of movement other
"than the blood and its animal spirits agitated by the heat
"of the fire which burns continually in the heart and which
"does not differ in nature from any of the other fires which
"are met with in inanimate bodies."

The prerogative of the rational soul is thought; the soul
understands, wishes, imagines, remembers and feels, for all
these are modes of thought; everything else is the work of
the bodily machine, sometimes actuated by the soul but sometimes not; and the soul always acts through the machine.
"The soul can call forth no movement in the body unless all
"the corporeal organs needed for the movement are properly
"disposed. On the other hand, when the body has all its
"organs properly arranged for a particular movement, it has
"no need of the soul to carry this out. Hence all movements
"except those which we know to depend upon thought ought
"not to be attributed to the soul but to the mere disposition
"of organs, and even the movements which we call voluntary
"depend principally on the same disposition of the organs
"(though it is the soul which is the determining cause) since
"without such a proper disposition we cannot carry them out,
"however much we will to do so. Because the movements
"cease when the body dies and the soul quits it, we must
"not therefore infer that it is the soul which produces them,
"since it is one and the same cause which on the one hand
"renders the body unfit to produce the movements and on
"the other hand leads the soul to quit the body."

If we judge Descartes from the severe standpoint of exact anatomical knowledge, we are bound to confess that he, to a large extent, introduced a fantastic and unreal anatomy in order to give clearness and point to his exposition. From this standpoint we cannot consider him as contributing to the progress of physiology; he stands in this respect wholly aside from Harvey or from other men of whom we are about to speak. On the other hand, however, we must admit that he did succeed in shewing that it was possible to apply to the interpretation not only of the physical but also of the psychical phenomena of the animal body, the same method which was making such astounding progress when applied to the phenomena of the material world. And indeed a very little change in the details of Descartes' exposition and some of that hardly more than a change in terminology would convert that exposition into a statement of modern views. If we read between the lines which he wrote, if we substitute in place of the subtle fluid of the animal spirits the molecular changes which we call a nervous impulse, if we replace his system of tubes with their valvular arrangements by the present system of concatenated neurons, whose linked arrangement determines the passage and the effects of the nervous impulses, Descartes' exposition will not appear so wholly different from the one which we give to-day.

Descartes was a philosopher, not a physiologist. He took interest in the problems of the living body only so far as they bore on the greater problems of the why and the wherefore of the universe. He entered into the details of vital functions and mingled in the controversies concerning them incidentally only, with the view of establishing or supporting his philosophical position. We must now turn back again to the physiologists proper.

Though Malpighi, as we have seen, devoted much attention to the histology of the nervous system, we find in his writings very little concerning its functions; and indeed an inquiry of a kind which must sooner or later lead the investigator into baseless speculations, and, at that time at least, any research into the properties of the nervous tissues seemed to be such, was wholly uncongenial to the character of his mind. Nor did this part of physiology appear to offer great attractions to many of the other men of the seventeenth century who were devoting themselves to exact anatomical and physiological research. One man alone perhaps during this century stands out prominently for his labours on the structure and functions of the brain, namely Thomas Willis.

Born at Great Bedwyn in Wiltshire on Jan. 27, 1621, Willis was educated at Oxford, where he took his M.A. degree in 1642. Remaining at Oxford, he was led in 1646, while that city was "garrisoned for the King," to employ his enforced leisure in the study of physic; and he eventually took up the profession of medicine. An enthusiastic royalist and staunch churchman, he was rewarded, upon the Restoration, by being made Sedleian Professor at Oxford; and for some years he was active there, practising his profession, fulfilling the duties of his Chair, and pursuing scientific researches. He was conspicuous among the band of men who in those years laid at Oxford the foundations of the Royal Society. In 1666 however he moved to London, "went," says Wood, "to the city "of Westminster, took a tenement in Saint Martin's Lane, "and in a very short time after he became so noted and so "infinitely resorted to, that never any physician before went "beyond him or got more money yearly than he. At length "after a great deal of drudgery that he did undergo in his "faculty (mostly for lucre sake) which did much shorten his "life, he concluded his last day in his house in Saint Martin's "Lane afore mentioned on the 11th day of November 1675."

Willis was not like Descartes a philosopher, and indeed was a man of a wholly different order; but he possessed what Descartes did not, a practical knowledge of the details of the structure and functions of the body and especially of the brain in health and disease. His work on the brain, by which our knowledge of cerebral structures was advanced far more largely than is indicated by the mere addition to anatomical nomenclature of the term 'circle of Willis,' became a classic work. The value of the book is indeed much above the worth of the author. Willis himself acknowledges that in his researches on the brain he was much assisted by Richard Lower; and Wood speaking of Lower says, "Willis "whom he helped or rather instructed." Lower as we have already seen was a real man of science, with a clear penetrating mind, with a genuine love of truth for truth's sake, a worthy mate of Boyle, of Hooke and of Mayow. Willis was of a different type; love of truth was in him less potent than love of fame. Mixing with and indeed in daily intercourse with the band of exact inquirers, who at Oxford and in London were striving to establish the new philosophy and advance by experiment natural knowledge, Willis caught up their phrases and, thinking himself one of them, attempted to expound in their fashion the physiology of the nervous system. But his method, when he was left to himself and deprived of the aid and guidance of Lower, was, in reality, wholly different from theirs. They made exact observations and careful experiments and, guided by the dry light of reason, drew conclusions with caution, and expounded them with brevity, using words only as expressing the meaning of things. Willis's mind was of the rhetorical sort, he loved words as words, looked upon an illustration as an argument, and when he discovered an analogy thought he had found a proof. Hence when we come to examine the views which he put forward, we find that while they are expounded with a certain philosophic air which perhaps goes far to explain the influence which they had in their time, they do not of themselves form any real solid contribution to knowledge. They are indeed to a large extent the views of Descartes, modified by more exact anatomical knowledge, occasionally by sound physiological deductions, in which we may probably trace the influence of Lower and other of Willis's contemporaries, but chiefly and especially by certain conceptions and certain modes of expression which appear to be entirely Willis's own.

He admits with Descartes that man possesses a rational soul, an immortal, incorporeal soul, but that, putting aside everything which is due to the direct activity of this rational soul, the nervous as well as the other phenomena both of man and of animals may be regarded as the phenomena of a corporeal machine. While, however, Descartes makes it his first object to prove that the body of man is, in this way, a machine, and that all known physiological phenomena may be adequately explained on this hypothesis, and has a secondary interest in physiological problems as such, caring for them only so long as they illustrate his thesis, Willis is especially concerned with these same special problems and in no case dwells on Descartes' main thesis.

Descartes speaks only of the animal spirits, accepting off-hand, as we have seen, the old views concerning them, but treating them from an exact physical point of view. Willis, in his rhetorical way, speaks of these animal spirits as con-stituting part of a corporeal soul, to whose activity are due the nervous phenomena of man and the higher animals; and he is especially concerned with the features and mode of action of this corporeal soul, this soul of the mere machine. He puts forward the view that this corporeal soul consists of two parts, one residing in the blood, the other in the brain and nervous system; and he believed that he had made a great discovery in recognizing the exact nature of these two parts of the soul. As I have said, Willis's mind was of that sort which when it has hit on an illustration or discovered an analogy, thinks it has found a proof. And the great dis-covery was simply this, that the part of the soul residing in the blood was of the nature of 'flame,' and the part residing in the brain and nervous system was of the nature of 'light.' This is what, in his rhetorical way, he says:

"The corporeal soul common to man and the higher "animals, while it extends over the whole organic body and "vivifies, actuates and irradiates every part, both tissues and "humours, yet seems more eminently to subsist in two of "these, and to hold them as its imperial seats as it were. "These subjects of the soul are on the one hand the vital fluid, "the blood, circulated in a perpetual round in the heart, "arteries and veins, and on the other the animal fluid or "nervous juice streaming gently through the brain and its "belongings. Both these provinces the soul inhabits and "adorns with its presence, but since the whole soul cannot "be in both provinces at the same time, it is as it were "divided, it actuates each province by its appropriate half. "One of its halves, since it is as we have shewn of the nature

"of fire, glides into the blood after the fashion of a lighted
"flame, while the other half seems diffused through the animal
"fluid after the manner of light, like the rays of light emanating
"from that flame, rays which, taken up by the brain and the
"nerves as by dioptic glasses and manifoldly reflected or
"refracted, form various figures according to the workings
"of the animal faculties.

"The animal soul therefore, corresponding to its dual chief
"functions in the animal body, consists of two distinct parts,
"namely, flame and light; for as regards the functions called
"natural, these are in truth only involuntary animal functions
"and are carried out by the aid of animal spirits."

He devotes a special treatise to prove that the blood is
aflame, is burning, that a flame exists in the blood. He had,
as I have said, many sound physiological views. He says of
the blood: "The functions of the blood at least in the higher
"animals are diverse and manifold. It instils into the brain
"and nervous system materials for the animal spirits, it
"provides nutritive juice for the various tissues, it supplies
"the elastic link to the motor structures, and besides secretes
"various residues and effete particles, and deposits them in
"the appropriate emunctories." Nor can even modern
physiology find fault with the following argument. "The
"following three things are especially essential requisites for
"the maintenance of a flame. In the first place a free and
"continuous access of air must be allowed to the flame so
"soon as it is lighted. In the second place the flame must
"enjoy a constant supply of sulphureous (combustible)
"material. In the third place the products of the flame
"whether gaseous or solid must be continually removed." All
these conditions are met with in the body. Fresh air is supplied
by breathing, sulphureous material is furnished by the food,
and the products of the flame in the blood are removed by
excretion through the skin.

He naturally finds a difficulty in the fact that the flame of
the blood is not visible; but this difficulty is not insuperable.

"But indeed the blood might be actually in flames and yet
"the light of it, on account of its tenuity, might not be visible
"to our eyes. We know that in the clear light of day we

"can see neither red-hot iron nor fireflies, nor ignes fatui nor "(phosphorescent) rotting wood, nor many other things which "are visible at night. Why then should not the vital fire, much "lighter than any of the above, escape our vision? Moreover "sometimes warm-blooded animals are wont to emit a visible "flame or fire at night only. For instance we have known "certain folk endowed with a warm and vaporous blood who "in the evening when on going to bed they take off their "underclothing near a fire or a candle, have emitted a very "delicate and shining flame which lit up all the lower parts "of their body. The cause of the above seems to be the same "as that by which a torch just put out and still smoking is "relighted by the merest trifle, shewing that a kind of flame, "the root of the one outside, lay hid in the torch. For the "same reason again the coats of horses, mules, cats and other "warm-blooded animals, when rubbed give rise to sparks "which in the dark may amount to a really conspicuous "light." And he goes on to quote the case of "an ingenious "man with an active brain who said that after an extra good "bout of wine he could see to read print clearly on a very "dark night."

Willis, as the above shews, had no great critical power in judging the value of evidence, and he was led to this idea of the flame of the blood, more by the force of the simile than by reasoning on facts; nevertheless, as the pupil of Harvey and as a comrade of the chemists of the day, he had laid hold of the view that the heat of the body is the heat of combustion, and in this respect was far above the old idea of the heat innate in the heart to which Descartes clung. He rejects this old idea in the words, "The heart gets its heat from the "blood, not the blood from the heart."

Having satisfied himself that the active properties of the blood, the vital spirits of the old teaching, are of the nature of flame, the same trust in the force of illustration led him to maintain that the active properties of the nervous system, the animal spirits, were of the nature of light.

"Although it is clear enough that such spirits are the "causes of animal functions and constitute the basis of the "soul itself, nevertheless it seems very difficult to explain

"what they are in their own proper essence, since scarcely
"anything occurs in nature with which in all respects they
"are comparable. The comparison of these with spirits of
"wine, of turpentine or of hartshorn, and the like, is by no
"means suitable. Besides that these chemical liquids neither
"represent the images of objects, nor exercise any elastic
"force, as do the animal spirits, they are moreover less subtle
"and volatile than these, since they can be poured or distilled
"from one vessel into another, whereas the animal spirits,
"vanishing directly that life is extinct, leave no trace of
"themselves behind. Wherefore we may far more rightly,
"according to our hypothesis, say that these spirits, emitted
"from the flame of the blood, are like rays of light, at least
"these joined with those of wind and air. For just as light
"is moulded to the impressions of all visible things, and air
"is moulded to the impressions of all audible things, so the
"animal spirits receive the images impressed on them, not
"only of the above, but also of odours and all tangible
"qualities, and deposit them in the common sensorium. But
"the air or aerial particles, so long as they are free and un-
"mixed, create no rush or tumult, yet when closely confined
"in clouds, or in machines, or brought into contact with
"sulphureous and other elastic corpuscles, being forthwith
"made wild, burst forth into often dreadful meteors, namely
"winds, whirlwinds and thunder. In the same way the animal
"spirits, so long as they are pure and are carried in the open
"spaces of the brain and its appendages, behave tranquilly
"enough, but when shut up within muscles, and these per-
"meated with sulphureous particles from the blood, and
"sometimes with heterogeneous matter in other places, be-
"come exceedingly impetuous, that is elastic, or spasmodic."

Though he hugged this idea of the animal spirits, the basis
of the corporeal soul, being of the nature of light, Willis was
no physicist. He caught up the phrases of his friends, Boyle
and others, without understanding them, and when he comes
to explain nervous phenomena, he mixes up the properties
of light with other physical phenomena, and indeed with
chemical phenomena. He speaks of the lighter, more spirituous
parts of the blood, as ascending by the carotid and vertebral

arteries, and as being distilled in the brain, and so prepared, as in a chemical operation, into animal spirits. These animal spirits are prepared in the cerebrum and cerebellum alone, in the cortex of each, and thence diffused over the whole nervous system. There are different kinds of animal spirits; those prepared in the cerebrum are destined for voluntary movement and sensation, those in the cerebellum for involuntary movements, for the beat of the heart, respiration and the like. These latter are simple, and have not the diversity of voluntary movements, hence the folds of the cerebellum, unlike those of the cerebrum, are all alike.

When, however, he discusses what we may call the general phenomena of nervous action he has recourse to the physical phenomena of fluids. The animal spirits pervade the whole nervous system, but in a special way. The nerves are not tubes along which the spirits flow, but solid fibres, and the animal spirits pass along them as spirits of wine pass along the stretched dry strings of a fiddle. This is how he explains nervous action:

"The internal and immediate efficient cause both of sense "and movement is furnished by the basis of the sensitive soul, "that is to say, by the animal spirits instilled into the brain "from the blood which is alight, and thence diffused into the "nervous system. These, being distributed by the brain, as "from a fount, along the nerves over the whole body, imbue, "irradiate, and fill all parts, inducing in each a certain tense- "ness. So that the ducts of the nervous structures, like cords "lightly strung, are extended from the brain and its append- "ages in every direction to all peripheral parts. And these "are so strung and so actuated by a certain continuity of the "soul (the corporeal soul), that if either extremity be struck, "the blow is forthwith felt throughout the whole. Hence any "intention conceived within the brain immediately carries "out the purposed work in the proper member or part, and "*vice versâ*, any impulse or blow which is inflicted from without "on any member or sensitive organ is immediately commu- "nicated to the brain. When the impression or impetus passes "outwards from the brain along the nerves to motor structures, "movement is produced. If on the other hand the impression

"started from without is carried inwards towards the brain,
"sensation is the result. While either of these is taking place,
"we must not suppose (as is commonly stated) that the same
"spirits rush at once from one goal to another as in a race-
"course or circus, and then rush back again; but since the
"soul by reason of a certain continuity is expanded over the
"whole, and its particles, that is to say the spirits, are
"arranged touching each other, drawn up as it were in line,
"so these, in military fashion, perform their functions, keep-
"ing their ranks without leaving their stations, and whether
"arranged in active fighting order, or passively as a mirror,
"themselves immobile, on the one hand obey the commands
"of the brain sent down from without, and so bring about
"movements, or on the other hand, pass straight on to the
"brain the message impressed on them by the sensitive
"structures, and thus give rise to sensation. So the same
"animal spirits bring about both movement and sensation,
"by their own opposite and inverse disposition and aspect."

And he explains diversity of functions by the argument,
"that it does not seem contrary to reason to suppose that
"within the basis of the sensitive soul and indeed within the
"same part of it, certain spirituous particles may be in
"movement while others remain at rest."

In the above Willis may be regarded as dimly striving to
explain nervous phenomena on the hypothesis of a specific
nervous fluid, possessed of peculiar properties, a kind of foreshadowing of an electric fluid. But when he comes to explain
the functions of the several cerebral structures he falls back
on his hypothesis of nervous action being light, or rather he
falls back on his illustration of light. Though the basis of the
sensitive soul, namely the animal spirits diffused through the
whole nervous system, is a physical, elastic fluid, the impressions on it which are developed into sensations are no
longer regarded as impulses, as in the passage which I quoted
just now, but as optic images.

The impressions made upon the sensory nerves by all
external objects pass through the middle parts of the brain,
through the crura cerebri to the corpora striata, thence to the
corpus callosum and so to the cortex. This is what he says:

"As regards the various functions and duties of the spirits "thus arranged in separate provinces, in the first place we "allot to them a twofold feature, one by which they work "inwards to carry on sensation, another by which they work "outwards to carry on movement. More particularly it seems "allowable to conceive of the middle regions of the brain as "constituting an inner chamber of this soul fitted with "dioptric mirrors, as with windows. The pictures or images of "all sensible things admitted into these secret places by means "of the ducts of the nerves, as by means of tubes or narrow "openings, first pass through the corpora striata, which "serves the purpose of an objective glass, and then are "represented on the corpus callosum as on a whitened wall. "And so the things which give rise to sensation induce "perception and a certain imagination. These images or "pictures thus formed there very often produce nothing but "the mere knowledge or sensation of the object, but presently "or at times having passed on, as it were by a second undula- "tion from the corpus callosum towards the cortex of the "brain, and being stored in its folds, give rise to the memory "of the thing, though the mere image vanishes. But if the "particular sensation impressed on the imagination gives "promise of something good or evil, forthwith the spirits "being excited, look back upon the object by whose impulse "they are set in motion, and for the sake of laying hold of it, "or of driving it away, very quickly delegate to other spirits "flowing along the ducts of the nerves, and so on to other "spirits of the members and of the motor parts, occupying "their proper places, the orders to carry out the appropriate "movements. Thus sense gives rise to imagination, this to "memory or to impulse, or to both of them, and impulse "finally gives rise to local movements, which bring about the "performance or the avoidance of the apparent good and "evil."

Thus all sensory nerves carry their impulses (as we now call them) to the corpora striata, which Willis repeatedly speaks of as the sensorium commune, the common seat of sensation, and produce further effects, first in the corpus callosum and then in the cortex. The same path is taken in the reverse direction by the motor impulses started by affections of mind. These also pass by the corpora striata, which Willis appears to have recognized as important organs no less of movement than of sensation; and his medical experience enabled him in many cases to connect disease in them with the symptoms of paralysis. We may add in passing that the same experience, as well as the results of his anatomical researches, led him to suppose that the optic thalamus was especially connected with sight.

I must not however tarry longer on Willis and his views; yet I cannot refrain from quoting one more passage which on the one hand shews that he had dimly laid hold of the modern doctrine of reflex action (and indeed other passages shew this), and on the other hand illustrates the difficulty which he met with in explaining all the phenomena of brute beasts by the mere possession of a material corporeal soul in the absence of that rational soul which belonged to man alone.

"We may admit that the impression of an object, driving "the animal spirits inwards, and modifying them in a certain "peculiar manner, gives rise to *sensation*, and that the same "animal spirits, in that they rebound from within outwards in "a reflected wave as it were, call forth *local movements*. We "have not, however, as yet stated how this soul or some part "of it *perceives that it feels*, and in accordance with that "*perception* is driven into various *passions* and *actions*, is "turned to the *desire* of this or that object, and sometimes, "as we may at times observe in certain beasts, in following "up the thing sought for, enters upon and carries out acts "which seem to have no other source than *judgment* and a "*certain deliberation*. Of course in man we can readily under-"stand that the *rational soul*, the governor as it were, looks "upon the images and impressions presented to the rational "soul as to a mirror, and according to the conceptions and "notions thus derived exercises the acts of *reason, judgment* "and *will*. In what way however in brute beasts, perception, "the discrimination of objects, desire, memory and other "forms of so to speak lower reason, are carried out seems very "difficult of explanation."

Willis's views did not escape severe criticism on the part of his contemporaries and even of his friends. John Mayow's strictly scientific spirit led him to apply to Willis's rhetorical expositions the following words:

"We have no need of I know not what vital flame by whose "deflagration the whole mass of the blood is heated, the heart "living like a salamander untouched in the midst of the "flames. Much less are we to suppose that such an intense "heating of the blood takes place as to be strong enough to "give rise to light, the rays of which, transmitted to the "brain, are to be thought to form the sensitive soul."

And again,

"As regards this lucid soul which dwells in the brains of "animals, I ask how it comes about that the light which is "supposed to illumine the whole brain and all the nerves can "never be seen by the eye? Assuredly Fires of this kind and "New Lights no less in Anatomy than in Religion appear to "me things wholly vain and fanatic."

The gifted Stensen also, in the remarkable lecture 'On the Anatomy of the Brain,' to which I have already referred, criticized very severely the views both of Descartes and of Willis. The burden of the lecture is that the anatomy of the brain is, for technical reasons, the most difficult part of all anatomy, and that, in spite of all that has been done, our knowledge of the real nature and disposition of the elements of the nervous system is most meagre.

"There abounds indeed a rich plenty of men to whom "everything is clear. Such, dogmatizing with the utmost "confidence, make up and publish the story of the brain and "the use of its several parts with the same assuredness as if "they had mastered with their actual eyes the structure of so ad- "mirable a machine and penetrated into the secrets of the great "artificer." Stensen perhaps especially directed this sarcasm against Descartes, whose merit as a philosopher, however, as we have seen, he duly recognized; but he doubtless had in his mind Willis also, with whose mere anatomy moreover he found fault, complaining of his figures as being inaccurate.

Stensen refused to admit, in face of the lack of all sound anatomical knowledge, any physiological deductions whatever.

After pointing out a number of cases in which he shews that adequate anatomical knowledge is wanting, he says, "whence "you may guess how little trust is to be put in explanations "based on such a futile foundation." "I have said nothing "of the use of parts, nothing of the actions which we call "animal, since it is impossible to explain the movements "carried out by a machine, so long as we remain ignorant "of the structure of its parts."

After pointing out the great difficulties which attend the dissection of the brain and especially all attempts in such tender structures to follow out the course and connections of the strands of fibres and other parts, he delivers himself of this pregnant passage:

"If indeed the white substance of which I am speaking "be, as in most places it seems to be, wholly fibrous in nature, "we must necessarily admit that the arrangement of its fibres "is made according to some definite pattern on which doubt- "less depends the diversity of sensations and movements." Had he, who in the earlier half of the seventeenth century thus foreshadowed the results of the last decades of the nineteenth century, been led to devote to the problems of the brain the same brilliant talents which had gathered in such valuable results in relation to glands and to muscle, the story of the progress of physiology of the nervous system in the times coming after him would, we may well think, have been very different from that which we have to record it actually is. But it was not to be. Stensen as we have seen was drawn to other things, and there was no one to take his place. After Willis a long period followed before anyone took up again the problems with which he had busied himself. Many valuable additions continued, it is true, to be made to the anatomy of the brain, slowly and from time to time; but for a long while no one took up the physiological inquiry with the fervour which had marked the middle of the seventeenth century. In tracing out the progress of science the trend of investiga- tion is found to vary from time to time; at one period men's minds are intently occupied with one set of problems, and at another period these seem to be without cause almost wholly neglected. But, even allowing for such an ill-understood rhythm of inquiry, it is difficult to resist the thought that the absence of research of which we are speaking was in part at least due to the sterilizing influence of Stahl's animistic doctrines.

During the eighteenth century, however, one remarkable advancement of knowledge was made, which, though it concerned not the functions of the brain proper, but the relations of the functions of nerves to those of muscle, had a remarkable influence over the whole of nervous physiology. This was the chief work of the great Haller, and to this we must now turn. In order, however, to appreciate the true value of Haller's labours it will be necessary even at the risk of some recapitulation to pass in review the various views put forward from time to time concerning the action of nerves, and the relation of that action to muscular movement.

In an early lecture I spoke of Borelli's ideas concerning muscular contraction and said a few words about his conception of nervous action. I must now return to these, especially the latter, and dwell upon some further details.

Borelli, as we saw, took a distinctly physical view of nervous action. To him the animal spirits were known as a succus nerveus, which he says "all recent authors admit is "not a breath (flatus) or air, but has a liquid consistency like "spirits of wine." This succus nerveus is agitated in two directions along the nerves, from the periphery to the brain as when it serves to generate sensations, and from the brain to the muscles as when it serves to give rise to movements. Acting in the latter direction it, as Willis also taught, performs a double function; it not only causes visible movements by means of the muscles, but also exercises a nutritive, plastic power by which in all the tissues the crude material furnished by the blood is fashioned into the living flesh.

He thus expounds the mechanical contrivance by which the spirituous juice (the succus nerveus) can, along the same nervous channels, be made to act both from without inwards, and from within outwards.

"The nerve fibres are," he says, "by no means solid, full "and impermeable, nor are they tubes hollow and empty like "reeds, but are canals filled with a certain spongy material

"like elder-pith. Such a marrow of the fibres can easily be
"moistened by the spirituous juice of the brain, to which it is
"conjoined, and may indeed be saturated to turgescence, as we
"see sponges are saturated by water in contact with them."

He uses as an illustration a sheep's intestine filled not with
water only, but with sponge impregnated with water, in which
a concussion at one end is in a moment communicated right
to the other end.

"In the same way, if one of the extremities of the nerve
"fibre be compressed or pushed, or struck or pinched, forth-
"with the commotion and concussion or undulation ought to
"be communicated right to the other end, because by reason
"of their contiguity, the parts lying first in an ordered series
"by pressing on those following, communicate the blow and
"the impulse right to the end.

"Hence it follows that the fibres or spongy ducts of certain
"nerves turgid with the spirituous juice can be shaken or
"pinched by that gentle motion of the spirits by which the
"acts of the command of the will are in the brain carried out,
"and then, by concussing the whole length of the nerve
"through the convulsive irritation, can squeeze out and dis-
"charge from their extreme orifices some spirituous droplets
"into the appropriate muscle, whence the ebullition and
"explosion follow by which the muscle is contracted and
"rendered tense.

"And on the other hand when the extremities of the sensory
"nerves which end in the skin, nose, ears or eyes, are com-
"pressed or struck or titillated, it necessarily follows that
"forthwith the concussion, undulation, or titillation of the
"spirituous juice contained within the tubules is conveyed
"along the whole length of the nerve and reaches the par-
"ticular part of the brain to which the nerve fibres are joined.
"And here the faculty of the sensitive soul according to the
"region of the brain thus percussed, according to the vehe-
"mence of the blow and the fashion and mode of the motion,
"is able to form a judgment concerning the object causing the
"movement."

He expressly declares that the "juices, however spirituous
"and active, are always corporeal and cannot act at a distance,

"and cannot, without physical contact, increase, intensify, or
"depress the animal spirits; it is by means of their corporeal
"presence that they either increase the animal spirits which
"are also corporeal, mixing themselves with them, or expel
"them, or transform them. Wherefore it cannot be conceived
"that nervous action can take place without some local
"movement of the nervous juice passing along the whole
"length of the nerve right to the brain."

Borelli's view of nervous action therefore was a strictly
physical one; in voluntary movement the concussion of the
nervous fluid started at the brain, and passing along the whole
length of the nerve, led to the ejection of some droplets of the
fluid into the substance of the muscle, and thus gave rise to
contraction. Of the act of contraction itself he was inclined
to take a chemical view, to believe that the inflation of a
muscle, which according to him was the essence of contraction,
was brought about "by something like a fermentation or an
"ebullition"; but of this he speaks guardedly.

Stensen, as we have seen, though he nowhere dwells on the
exact nature of nervous action or its relation to muscular
contraction, had arrived at conceptions of the nature of
muscular contraction itself, more true and exact than those
even of Borelli. He laid hold more clearly than Borelli seems
to have done of the truth that the contraction of a muscle
is the result of the contraction of the individual fibres; and
he quotes the experiment that when a long muscle is cut up
lengthways by scissors in three or four bits, each bit may be
made to contract, as a proof that the power of contraction
resides in the muscular substance as substance and not in
the whole muscle as a machine. He further states that
contraction is not dependent on the action of arteries, or
veins, or even necessarily on that of nerves; and he insists
that while all voluntary movement is brought about by
muscles, every movement which a muscle carries out is not
necessarily a voluntary one. He ends his essay on muscle
with the following remarkable speculation:

"Concerning the fluid of muscles how uncertain, or rather
"how wholly wanting, is our knowledge. Fluid certainly exists
"in the fibrillae of which the motor fibres are composed and

"between the fibrillae, also between the motor fibres them-
"selves, in the membranous fibrillae" (that is the connective
tissue), "and between the membranous fibrillae; but in truth
"it is by no means clear whether these fluids are all of one
"kind or whether just as they are distinct in the seats which
"they occupy so they differ in material properties.

"Nor is it known whether any of these fluids are really like
"any one of the fluids so far known to us. Animal spirits, the
"more subtle part of the blood, the vapour of blood, and the
"juice of the nerves, these are names used by many, but they
"are mere words, meaning nothing. Some going further bring
"forward saline and sulphureous particles or something
"analogous to spirits of wine. Such things may perhaps be
"true, but are neither certain nor adequately distinct. Ex-
"perience teaches us that a dose of spirits of wine restores
"exhausted powers, but who shall have determined whether
"that which restores the fluid spirit is to be ascribed to this
"said humour which we call spirit or to some other material
"or is joined to it through some other cause?

"As the substance of this fluid is unknown to us, so is its
"movement undetermined, since neither by sure reasoning
"nor by experiment has it been ascertained whence it comes,
"whither it tends, where on its departure it betakes itself.

*   *   *   *   *

"There remains another difficulty of no less moment not
"yet cleared up, namely in what respect the movement of the
"fluid in a muscle while it is contracting differs from the
"movement of the fluid in the same muscle when it remains
"quiet, uncontracted. Is its quantity changed? or does it
"remain the same? Is the fluid after the event, supposing it
"remains, the same as before the event? Does the fluid move
"because the muscle contracts, or does the contraction of the
"solid proceed from the movement of the fluid?"

This singular man had three hundred years ago pierced into
questions which are still moving us at the present day.

Since this is the last occasion which I shall have to speak
of Stensen, I may here venture to quote his appeal on behalf
of the value of science in practical matters:

"It may be shewn abundantly elsewhere how much medical
"practice owes to the anatomical experiments of this age, even
"if it were only for this that they have exposed the numerous
"errors which occur in the explanation of the causes of disease
"and at the same time shewn the reasons which have governed
"the application of remedies to be in most cases erroneous.
"To those who decry the value of science I would give as an
"answer this demand that they should ask their own con-
"sciences and see what solid basis there is for all those
"dogmas which they pronounce with such bold ease when
"they explain the symptoms of apoplexy, paralysis, con-
"vulsions, prostration of strength, syncope, and other diseases
"affecting animal movements, on what foundation they rest
"when they apply remedies for removing these evils, with
"the result that they do away not with the paralysis, not
"with the convulsion, but with the paralytic or the convulsed
"man."

Willis was very far from reaching the exact standpoint of
Borelli and Stensen; he explains muscular contraction in a
very different way. This is what he says:

"The animal spirits carried from the brain by the channels
"of the nerves to a muscle, caught up by the membranaceous
"fibrillae, and carried by means of these to the fibres of the
"tendon, are then plenteously stored up as it were in suitable
"storehouses. These spirits, being by nature exceedingly
"active and elastic, upon expanding as their power and
"opportunity permit, leap into the fleshy fibres, and presently
"afterwards, their impetus being exhausted, falling back,
"they retreat again into the tendons; and this is repeated
"again and again. When however the animal spirits at the
"bidding of the instinct to bring about movement rush from
"the tendinous to the fleshy fibres, they there meet with
"active particles of a different nature supplied by the blood,
"and forthwith the two mixing, effervesce, so that out of the
"struggle and agitation of the two, the fleshy fibres, previously
"lax and porous, are stuffed full and thrown into corrugations,
"and all the fibres being thus corrugated at the same time,
"the contraction of the whole muscle is brought about. The
'contraction being finished, the pure spirits which remain

"for the most part retreat again into the tendinous fibres,
"the remaining particles being left among the fleshy fibres.
"The loss which has occurred among the latter is made good
"by the blood, that among the former by the nerves."

Mayow, as we have seen, had his own view about the matter
in question. He like many other discoverers who have laid
hold of a great truth, but have not had time to go all round it,
was inclined to see in his spiritus nitro-aereus an explanation
of nearly all the unexplained phenomena of the universe;
he used it to explain muscular contraction. This was in his
view a fermentation set up between the combustible, sulphureous particles residing in the muscle, and the nitro-aereal
spirit brought to it by the nerves. But he got no further than
this.

While these several men of the seventeenth century whom
I have just mentioned were hovering about the truth of the
relation of nervous influences to muscular contraction, some
getting more, others less near, one among them, an Englishman, came upon the truth itself, and after him this part of
physiology stood still for near a hundred years. This was
Francis Glisson, of whom I have already said something more
than once, but of whom I must now speak in more detail.

Born in 1597 at Rampisham in Dorset of a good family,
Glisson entered in 1617 as a scholar at Gonville and Caius
College, Cambridge, where for a while he threw himself with
vigour and success into the usual learning of the place, taking
office in his college in 1624 as Fellow, in 1625 as Lecturer on
Greek, and in 1629 as Dean, though not in holy orders. Later
on, the publication of Harvey's work in 1628 being possibly
the determining cause, he turned his mind to medicine, and
becoming in 1634 Doctor of Medicine was in 1636 appointed
Regius Professor of Physic. He appears to have carried out
his medical studies in London, for there is no evidence of his
ever having like Harvey gone abroad. Though for some time
he practised as a physician in Colchester, the greater part of
his life was passed in London, where he was very active at
the College of Physicians, of which he became Fellow in 1635,
and Reader in Anatomy in 1639. He was one of the small
band of men who used to meet in 1660 at Gresham College

to discuss natural knowledge, and who two years later founded
the Royal Society. He seems to have spent very little time
at Cambridge, treating his professional duties somewhat
lightly. Though he held his Chair until his death, Dr Brady
being appointed his deputy in 1675, there is no evidence of his
ever having delivered any courses of lectures; yet he appears
to have attended at Cambridge from time to time "to keep
acts" when candidates presented themselves for the degree
of Doctor of Medicine. In 1650 he petitioned the University
for five years' arrears of salary, apparently the years 1643–4
to 1648–9, when, living at Colchester, he was wholly absent.
Probably life at Cambridge was distasteful to him; the
University was very strongly Royalist, and Glisson was a pronounced Presbyterian. While at Colchester he served as elder
of the church at the neighbouring village of Lexden; and
being shut up in 1648 in Colchester with the Royalists in the
memorable siege of that place, was chosen by the besieged
authorities as a very suitable member of the deputation sent
forth to treat with Fairfax on the terms of surrender. While
in London he did his duties manfully during the great plague
of 1665, was President of the College of Physicians 1667–9,
and passed away at a ripe old age in 1677.

He was a good anatomist and a sound physician; and he is
perhaps best known for his classic works on rickets and on the
liver. With the latter I have dealt in speaking of Malpighi.
Yet the work to which he gave most of his energy, and the
one which best illustrates the character of his mind, is the
Tractatus de natura substantiae energetica, published in 1672
when he was an old man. For, accurate and careful anatomist
though he was, Glisson was essentially a philosopher, steeped
in all the old Aristotelean learning which he had eagerly
devoured in his youth, and striving to shape that old learning
into accordance with the new philosophy which was fermenting around him. The *Tractatus* in fact is a bold attempt
to shew that all phenomena as well as of living things, be they
animal or vegetable, as of things not alive, are the successive
developments of the one fundamental energy of nature. He
says of this work in his preface, "It treats of Nature, well
"known by name but really understood by few, that Nature

"of which so many splendid things have been said by ancient
"as well as modern Philosophers. But the few who have so
"far recognized this life of nature have neither made clear its
"substantial origin in material things nor adequately dis-
"tinguished it from vegetable or animal life. Still less have
"they, following up its more hidden traces, inquired how it is
"developed from the natural into the vegetable and animal.
"Least of all have they shewn how the material soul, the
"vegetative soul and the sensitive soul arise out of the life
"of nature, though this is lifted up by successive steps."

He confesses that he has done no more than sketch out
the *à priori* proof of his view. The *à posteriori* proof has only
just been begun. That can not be supplied by an old man like
himself or indeed by the hands of any one man. "Let me
"hope that the Royal Society and other inquirers after truth
"will be moved to furnish it."

I call attention to this general view of Glisson's, because
this was the mother idea which led him to a special conception
of the properties of muscular tissue, through which he
anticipated modern teaching by nearly a hundred years. In
his work on the liver, in discussing how it comes about that
the bile is discharged into the intestines at certain times only,
namely when it is wanted, he shews that the gall-bladder and
biliary duct bring about a greater excretion when they are
irritated. And he argues that they cannot be irritated unless
they possess the power of being irritated. This power of being
irritated he proposes to denote by the term *irritability*. And
he develops this view again in his work on the stomach, *De
Ventriculo*, published the year of his death, though wholly
written as early as 1662, but laid aside in order that he might
devote himself to his work *De Natura*.

Thus it is undoubtedly to Glisson that we owe the first
introduction not only of the word but of the idea of 'irritability,' which, revived by Haller, as we shall immediately see,
in the next century, became firmly established in physiology,
and has played an important part in the development both
of physiological and pathological views. Haller used the
word in its narrower sense as the property through which
muscle responds by movement to an external stimulus; since

then it has been extended to mean response in any way, not by movement or change of form only but by any kind of change, chemical change, change of growth, and the like. And it is worthy of note that Glisson from the very first used the word in its widest sense, distinguishing the various ways in which irritability may be manifested and the various agents by which it may be called forth.

It was perhaps by reason of the fundamental and highly philosophic character of Glisson's conception that it did not meet with immediate recognition. The idea had to be put forth in the narrower form, which Haller gave to it, in order to be understood and accepted by physiological people.

Besides this introduction of the idea of irritability Glisson made another contribution to muscular physiology of a wholly different character, and yet one, from another point of view, of fundamental importance. We have seen that Borelli, with all his zeal for the exact mathematical treatment of physiological problems, assumed, being led to do so by reasons of analogy, without attempting to make any direct observations on the matter, that a muscle during contraction was inflated, that it suffered increase in bulk. Now Borelli took this view although as we have seen he had freed himself from the old, and to a large extent still current grosser conceptions of the nature of the animal spirits. To those who held these grosser conceptions the increase in bulk of a muscle during its contraction was a natural and indeed necessary postulate; the animal spirits flowed into the muscle and made it swell up. Such, with the admixture of certain new chemical conceptions, was as we have seen the teaching of Willis.

All such ideas Glisson confronted with a single experiment, the result of which deprived them of all solid basis. He gave, and he was the first to give, the exact proof that when a muscle contracts it does not increase in bulk; and his old experiment still stands in substance as the proof given in our modern text-books. In his work *De Ventriculo* he says:

"But indeed this explosion and inflation of spirits has now "for some time past been silenced, convicted by the following "experiment. Take an oblong glass tube of suitable capacity "and shape. Fit into the top of its side near its mouth

"another small tube like a funnel. Let a strong muscular
"man insert into the mouth of the larger tube the whole of
"his bared arm, and secure the mouth of the tube all round
"to the humerus with bandages so that no water can escape
"from the tube. Then pour water through the funnel until
"the whole of the larger tube is completely filled, and some
"water rises up into the funnel. This being done, now tell
"the man alternately to contract powerfully and to relax the
"muscles of his arm. It will be seen that when the muscles
"are contracted the water in the tube of the funnel sinks,
"rising again when relaxation takes place. From which it is
"clear that muscles are not inflated or swollen at the time
"that they are contracting, but on the contrary are lessened,
"shrunk, and subsided. For if they were inflated the water
"in the tubule so far from sinking would rise. From this
"therefore we may infer that the fibres are shortened by an
"intrinsic vital movement and have no need of any abundant
"afflux of spirits, either animal or vital, by which they are
"inflated, and being so shortened carry out the movements
"ordered by the brain."

We nowadays avoid the concomitant changes in the volume
of blood present in the arm, and take not a whole limb of
man but the bloodless muscles of a frog; but otherwise the
plethysmographic proof we now use is identical with that of
Glisson.

But Glisson's irritability and his notable experiment were
like Mayow's igneo-aereal spirit forgotten as the seventeenth
century passed into the eighteenth. We have to wait until the
middle of the latter century, when the truth was brought to
light again by the sagacious Haller in his views of nervous
action and its relation to muscular contraction. To these we
must now turn.

In his *Elementa*, Haller in treating of the subject begins by
discussing the contractile force in general. "There is widely
"present not only in the animal but also in the vegetable
"kingdom a contractile force by which the elements of fibres
"are brought nearer to each other. This not only seems to be
"the cause of cohesion in general, but is rendered manifest
"by the fact that a fibre drawn out lengthways when let go

"very soon returns to its previous length, and never lays
"aside the effort to become shorter until it has so returned
"to its previous length." This is more properly the elastic
force. Besides this there is a contractile force by which the
tissues dead or alive shrink when treated in various ways,
when for instance they are heated. A contractile force of such
a kind is present in almost all animal tissues, unless it be the
very soft and pulpy ones like brain or the very hard ones like
bone and teeth. But there is in addition a special contractile
force proper to muscles alone. "In a living animal, or in one
"only just dead, there very frequently appears spontaneously
"in muscular tissue a swift vivid contractile movement by
"which the ends of the muscle are alternately brought nearer
"to the middle belly and then again recede from it." And
even when this contractile movement does not spontaneously
appear, it may be excited if a stimulus, such as pricking, or
pinching, or some chemical substance be applied.

Many writers consider this living contractile force as identical with the dead one just described as belonging more or
less to all tissues. This view Haller discusses and concludes,
"that muscular fibre is the only one which is moved spon-
"taneously in the living animal, or is brought by irritaments
"from rest to movement," and that "the living contractile
"force must be held to be distinct from the dead contractile
"force, since the two agree neither in the laws which govern
"them, nor in their duration, nor in their seat."

This force he calls the *vis insita*, the 'inherent force,' and
the tissues possessing it he calls after Glisson 'irritable.'

He then discusses whether this property of irritability is
identical with that of feeling, and concludes that it is not.
"There are many parts which feel but which are not
"irritable, and in particular a nerve, which is above every-
"thing sensitive, and yet possesses no contractile force ex-
"cept that common one found as stated above even in dead
"things.

"Wherefore this force since it is different both from mere
"elasticity and from that dead contraction which is common
"to all fibres, seems to constitute a peculiar property, proper
"to the muscular fibre, and indeed to mark the character of

"that fibre, so that every muscular fibre is irritable, and on
"the other hand you may fairly call muscular fibre every-
"thing that is irritable. It is however a force of its own kind,
"different from every other power, and to be classed among
"the sources of the production of motion the ultimate cause
"of which is unknown. This same force is inherent in the fibre
"itself and not brought to it from without."

He sums up thus:

"I (by my experiments published first in 1739, and again
"in 1743) separated this irritable nature on the one hand
"from a mere dead force, and on the other from the nervous
"force and from the power of the soul. I shewed that the
"movement of the heart and the irritable nature of the
"intestines depended on it alone. I confined it entirely to
"the muscular fibre, in which point the Batavian school does
"not agree with me, but they will I hope do so when they are
"willing to distinguish the contractile force common to all
"animal fibre from the irritable force proper to muscle alone.
"I also shewed that that force was something perpetually
"living, and that it often broke out into movement though
"no external stimulus such as could be recognized by us was
"acting. By a stimulus, however, it could at any time be
"called back from rest into action. In a movement produced
"through it I distinguished between the stimulus which
"might be very slight, and the movement called forth by
"the stimulus which might be very powerful."

"Some," says he, "have wished to call this force the vital
"force, but this does not quite please me since the force may
"for some little time survive the life of the body. Hence I
"prefer to call it the force inherent in or proper to muscle."
He then goes on:

"Besides this force inherent in muscular fibre, another force
"is exercised in it, so far like the former in that it alone has
"its seat in muscular fibre. But it is different from the in-
"herent force in as much as it comes from without and is
"carried to the muscles from the brain by the nerves, it is
"the power by which muscles are called into action." This he
calls the *vis nervosa*. It too survives the death of the body,
and in cold-blooded animals is of the same constancy as the

inherent force, so that in such an animal recently killed, in which no sensation or voluntary movement remains, a muscle, provided it be moist and whole, is thrown into convulsions when its nerve is irritated. And the same is true of warm-blooded animals.

Having thus cleared the way by adopting the conception that the movements of the body are the manifestations of this inherent contractile power of muscle, the *vis insita*, which may develop itself spontaneously, but which is usually brought into play by the instrumentality of the nerves, by the *vis nervosa*, Haller was able, in his remarkable chapter, 'On the Phenomena of the living Brain,' to deal in a true scientific spirit, indeed in a modern spirit, with the many and difficult problems of the nervous system.

He first confines himself to what can be learnt from experiment. "As the nature of the brain and of the nerves is one "and the same, so are these alike in function. In treating "of them we will so far as possible make use of experiments, "nor will we at first at least go beyond the testimony of our "senses."

Experiments and the testimony of the senses teach us, he says, that nerves alone feel: only those parts which possess nerves feel, and they feel through their nerves. The question whether tendons feel presented difficulties to him as it has done to others after him; but the main result of all his experiments confirmed him in the view that nerves are the only instruments of sensation, just as they by calling into play the contractile power of muscles are the only instruments of movement.

All the nerves are gathered together into the 'medulla cerebri,' into the central parts of the brain; whence it may be inferred that "this central part of the brain feels and that in "it are presented to the mind the impressions which the "nerves disturbed at their extreme ends have carried to the "brain." This conclusion is supported by the phenomena of disease and by the results of experiments on living animals. Sensation manifests itself by movements, and when these central parts of the brain are irritated by the knife or otherwise, the movements which follow abundantly prove that

sensation has been excited. These movements are readily seen
when the corpora striata, the thalamus, the crura cerebri,
the pons and the medulla oblongata are injured. He goes on
to argue that the cortex of the brain must also feel, though
no movement results when it is irritated. "But the medulla
"of the corpora striata, or of the crura, or of the pons differs
"in no way from that of the rest of the brain except the actual
"cortex, and this unless it itself felt would be unable to bestow
"feeling on the medulla. If indeed the medulla is one and
"the same, and exactly alike at the summit and at the base
"of the brain, and if the deeper medulla obviously feels, it
"cannot with any right be said that the medulla placed in the
"higher situation, though possessing exactly the same nature,
"is destitute of feeling. The nerves therefore feel and carry
"to the brain the impressions of external objects. Those im-
"pressions are preserved in the brain, and after fifty or even
"after a hundred years, if a man lives so long, remain vivid
"and clear."

He then goes on to discuss the question whether any
particular parts of the brain, by a special privilege, function
as the seat of sensation and the source of movement. "In all
"cases we have shewn that the impressions of the senses are
"carried to the brain, and the cause of movement is con-
"veyed thence through the nerves to the muscles of the whole
"body. But learned men, even those of the school of Galen
"as well as those of recent years, have suspected that the
"power of receiving feeling and of exciting movement was not
"alike in particular parts of the brain, and that the whole
"brain was not necessary for the full development of sensa-
"tions." He discusses this question, using as tests the phenomena of disease and the results of experiments on animals.
Guided by these, he rejects the view held by Willis and others
that the corpora striata serve as the seat of sensation and the
source of movement, as well as the view that the cerebellum
is essential to life. In the light of our modern knowledge it is
most interesting to follow this physiologist of a hundred and
fifty years ago striving to find his way along the tangled path
presented by the nervous phenomena resulting from disease
or from experimental interference.

He then passes on to what he calls 'conjectures.' The views which he has "so far put forward have been based on the "evidence of the senses, and if we have erred the error has lain "in the experiment. This fault however can readily be mended "since by simple repetition it can be ascertained whether we "are really following nature's lead or have wandered from the "truth, led astray by the fewness of the experiments or by "some mistake in carrying them out. It is not equally easy "to keep oneself from error in the matters which have now "to be discussed. Very little of what follows is based on the "evidence of the senses, but is reached by probable arguments "gathered from all manner of sources, and these while they "are strong enough to furnish ourselves with the hope of "truth, do not possess that certainty which will carry con-"viction to the mind of others."

The first subject which he discusses, 'by conjectures,' is the nature of nervous action. He expounds and rejects the view put forward under various shapes that the nerves act as solid bodies, after the fashion, for instance, of elastic strings along which vibrations are conveyed. In his encyclopaedic manner he recalls and discusses various views of this kind put forward by various men, including that of Nicolas Robinson, who in his work on the spleen supposed that the nerves of sense were composed of little papillary machines, exceedingly small and exceedingly numerous and minute, which struck by the object giving rise to the sensation were thrown into oscillations and so conveyed the impression to the mind.

He next discusses the view that nervous action depends upon a fluid.

"All the ancients attributed to the nerves a most subtle and "attenuated humour or rather fluid, for the word humour "suggests something sluggish, to which they gave the name "of spirits, and which, though invisible just like air, exercises "a great power. This doctrine of the schools for many ages "held its place; lately, however, this doctrine of spirits, like "all other things which pleased of old, began to totter. Then "a sect by no means weak" (namely that of Stahl) "took up "the position that the soul acted directly hand to hand in all "the actions of the body and did not make use of instruments, "by which it conveyed its commands to distant parts. People "began to doubt very much about these spirits, and indeed "now even the most distinguished men share these doubts."

He first marshals all that can be said against this hypothesis of the spirits, that is of the active part of the nerve being of the nature of a fluid, quoting among other things the argument that a nerve when ligatured does not swell, and the like. But he finds these objections invalid; and assuming therefore that the active nervous material is of a fluid nature, he proceeds to discuss what must be its essential characters. These lead him to the conclusion that it cannot be of the nature of an albuminous solution, nor spirituous in nature like alcohol, nor acid, nor sulphureous, *i.e.* combustible. He likewise decides that it cannot be, as so many have thought, aerial. "At the close of the seventeenth century," he says, "the "name ether came into fashion, and it became the wont to "attribute to it, to an invisible element which did not lend "itself to experiment, everything the cause of which was "unknown, light, gravity, magnetism. Some accordingly hold "the spirits (the nervous fluid) to be of the nature of ether "or to be composed of ether." He rejects this also, including in the rejection the view that the spirits consist of electric material.

"Of what nature then," he asks, "is the material of these "spirits?" He answers, with the spirit of the eclectic philosopher that he was, "an element of its own kind unlike "everything else. An element, too subtle to be grasped by "any of the senses, but more gross than fire, or ether or "electric or magnetic matter, since it can be contained in "channels and restrained by bonds and moreover is clearly "produced out of and nourished by food. What forbids, since "light is something different from fire, and the material of "the magnet differs from both, and air and ether are unlike "all the rest, what forbids that there should be this element "of its own kind known to us only by its effects?"

He then discusses as a speculation, but be it observed as a speculation only, whether the nerves are hollow for the conveyance of this nervous fluid; he decides in the affirmative and insists that by analogy the fibres of the brain must in like manner be hollow also. He adds that the nervous fluid is supplied and nourished by the arteries of the brain.

He rejects the view of there being two different kinds of nervous fluid, one for the production of sensation and movement, and another for the preservation of life, one connected with the cerebrum, the other with the cerebellum. He rejects also the view that there is one kind of nervous fluid for sensation and another for movement; he sees no real difficulty in the same nerve serving both for sensation and movement.

Lastly, he passes to the most speculative question of all, the 'seat of the soul.' He rejects the Stahlian opinion that the soul and the sensorium commune is diffused over the whole body, present as well in the tip of the finger as in the brain. He recalls the results arrived at by experiment that the medulla, the central part of the brain, is the seat of sensation and the source of muscular movement. "Nor in "the cortex of the brain alone is the seat of sensation or "the full origin of the cause of muscular movement; each of "these lies also in the medulla of the cerebrum and of the "cerebellum." "This is not the place to speak about the "soul, but the soul has nothing in common with the body "other than sensation and movement. Now both sensation "and movement have their source in the medulla of the "brain. This therefore is the seat of the soul."

Asking the question whether the seat of the soul can be defined within narrower limits, he remarks that "no narrower "seat can be allotted to the soul than the conjoint origin of "all the nerves; nor can any structure be proposed as its seat "except that to which we can trace all the nerves. For it will "be easily understood that the sensorium commune ought to "lack no feeling of any part of the whole animated body nor "any nerve which can convey from any part of the body the "impression of external objects. And the same may be said "of the nerves of movement. Wherefore, even quite apart "from the experimental results described above, we cannot "admit as the exclusive seat of the soul, either the corpus "callosum or the septum lucidum or the tiny pineal gland, "or the corpora striata or any particular region of the "brain."

There remains still a somewhat different question whether different parts of the brain may not correspond to different functions of the soul. Some experiments and some of the phenomena of disease do, he admits, give a certain support to this, and the anatomical evidence points in the same direction; we may for instance suppose that the parts of the brain around the entrance of the optic nerve are especially concerned in vision, and the like. We may perhaps go a certain way in this direction, but a very little way. "Our "present knowledge does not permit us to speak with any "show of truth about the more complicated functions of the "mind or to assign in the brain to imagination its seat, to "common sensation its seat, to memory its seat. Hypotheses "of this kind have in great numbers reigned in the writings "of physiologists from all time. But all of them alike have "been feeble, fleeting, and of a short life."

Thus Haller wrote in the middle of the eighteenth century. The nineteenth century has brought great gains to our knowledge of the nervous system. Charles Bell and Majendie laid bare to us that fundamental distinction between sensory and motor fibres which Haller failed to see. The hidden work of the vaso-motor nerves, and of the other nerves which answer to calls not those of the will, and which often play their parts in silence without awakening consciousness, has been revealed to us. The progress of physical and especially of electric science has given us conceptions of how the pulses of sense and of the will fly inwards and outwards along the nerve-fibres, conceptions clear and definite compared with Haller's dim gropings after the nature of the nervous fluid. And above all in these later years, the microscopical study, by refined methods, of healthy and especially of diseased nervous structures, carried out in concert with exact experiments on living animals have gathered for us knowledge concerning those different provinces of the brain which serve the different functions of the mind—knowledge clear, definite, and founded on fact in place of Haller's timorous conjectures, and have brought us within measurable distance of being able to assign, not as feeble, short-lived hypotheses, but as proved experimental results, to sensation its seat, to memory its seat, and even to imagination its seat. We have learnt much since Haller's time. But what I have said of Haller justifies, I venture to think, the assertion that we have gone forward so much because we have laboured on Haller's lines. He expounded the nervous system in a spirit which has become the modern spirit, and our progress has been due to our following his example. And if he with the knowledge and the means at his command seems to us to-day often to have walked haltingly or even often to have gone astray, we may ask ourselves this question: Are not we, with all the knowledge and the means at our command, walking also haltingly, if not more haltingly; and are we not as often, if not more often, going astray? Shall we not seem so to those who tell our story a hundred years to come? For indeed it is one of the lessons of the history of science that each age steps on the shoulders of the ages which have gone before. The value of each age is not its own, but is in part, in large part, a debt to its forerunners. And this age of ours if, like its predecessors, it can boast of something of which it is proud, would, could it read the future, doubtless find also much of which it would be ashamed.

A CHRONOLOGICAL TABLE OF THE CHIEF WRITERS
SPOKEN OF IN THE FOREGOING LECTURES

Name	Birthplace	Birth	Death	Title and Date of Chief physiological or anatomical Work	
Mundinus	Bologna		1326	De Anatome	1315
Berengarius, Jacobus (Carpi)	Carpi	1470	1530	Commentaria	1521
Guinterius, Johannes	Andernach	1487	1574	Institutiones Anatomicae	1536
Paracelsus (Theophrastus von Hohenheim)	Einsiedeln	1490	1541	Chirurgia Magna	1536
Sylvius, Jacobus	Amiens	1478	1555	Commentarium	1539
Vesalius, Andreas	Brussels	1514	1564	Fabrica Humani Corporis	1543
Servetus, Michael	Villanueva	1511	1553	Christianismi Restitutio	1553
Columbus, Matheus Realdus	Cremona	1516	1559	De Re Anatomica	1559
Falloppius, Gabrielus	Modena	1523	1563	Observationes Anatomicae	1561
Caesalpinus, Andreas	Arezzo	1519	1603	Quaestiones Peripateticae	1571
Fabricius, Hieronymus	Aquapendente	1537	1619	De Venarum ostiolis	1574
Sanctorius, Sanctorius	Capo d'Istria	1561	1636	Statica Medica	1614
Aselli, Gaspar	Cremona		1626	De Lactibus	1627
Harvey, William	Folkestone	1578	1667	Exercitatio de Cordis motu	1628
Van Helmont, Jean Baptiste	Brussels	1577	1644	Ortus Medicinae	1648
Pecquet, Jean	Dieppe	1624	1674	Experimenta Nova Anatomica	1651
Glisson, Francis	Rampisham	1597	1677	De Hepate	1654
Wharton, Thomas	Winston-on-Tees	1614	1673	Adenographia	1656
Willis, Thomas	Great Bedwyn	1621	1666	Cerebri Anatome	1659
Boyle, Robert	Lismore	1627	1691	New Experiments physico-mechanical	1660
Malpighi, Marcello	Crevalcore	1628	1694	De Pulmonibus	1661
Bellini, Lorenzo	Florence	1643	1703	De Structura Renum	1662
Descartes, René	Tours	1596	1650	De Homine Liber	1662
Stensen, Nicolas	Copenhagen	1638	1686	Observationes Anatomicae	1662
Sylvius, Franciscus	Hanover	1614	1672	Disputationes	1663
De Graaf, Regnier	Schoonhoven	1641	1673	De Natura et usu succi pancreatici	1664

Name	Birthplace	Birth	Death	Title and Date of Chief physiological or anatomical Work	
Hooke, Robert	Freshwater	1635	1703	Micrographia	1667
Mayow, John	London	1643	1679	De Sal Nitro, etc.	1668
Lower, Richard	Cornwall	1631	1690	Tractatus de Corde	1669
Peyer, Jean Conrad	Schaffhausen	1653	1712	De Glandulis Intesti-norum	1677
Borelli, Giovanni Alphonso	Naples	1608	1679	De Motu Animalium	1680–1
Brunner, Jean Conrad	Diessenhofen	1653	1727	Experimenta nova circa pancreas	1682
Stahl, Georg Ernest	Anspach	1660	1734	Theoria Medica	1708
Boerhaave, Hermann	Voorhout	1668	1738	Institutiones Medicae	1708
Reaumur, René Antoine Ferchault	Rochelle	1683	1757	Sur la Digestion	1752
Black, Joseph	Bordeaux	1728	1799	De Humore Acido	1754
Haller, Albrecht	Bern	1708	1777	Elementa Physiologiae	1757
Priestley, Joseph	Fieldhead	1733	1804	Experiments and Observations on different Kinds of Air	1775–7
Lavoisier	Paris	1743	1794	Sur la nature du principe	1775
Spallanzani, Lazaro	Scandiano	1729	1799	Dissertazioni di fisica animale e vegetabile	1783

INDEX

Academia del Cimento, 63
Academy of Sciences, suppression of, by the Convention, 252
'Acini,' the, of Malpighi, 111, 112
Albinus, Frederick Bernard, Professor of Anatomy at Leyden, 203
Alimentary canal, 47, 51
'Animism,' Stahl the founder of, 171
Archaeus, the, 124, 126, 130, 134, 137, 141, 166, 167
Artery-like vein, 11, 22, 28, 32, 38, 39, 43, 58, 94
Aselli, Gaspar, the discoverer of the lacteals, 48–51, 129, 137; 'pancreas of Aselli,' 49

Bacon, Francis, *Novum Organon* of, 129
Bassi, Laura, holds the Chair of Mathematics at Bologna, 210
Beccher, Johann Joachim, the *Physica subterranea* of, 166; *Specimen Beccherianum* of Sylvius, 166
Bell, Charles, on sensory and motor fibres, 296
Bellini, Laurentio, the *Structura renum* of, 109; Professor of Anatomy at Pisa, *ib.*; physician to Cosimo III, 109
Bentley, Richard, establishes an 'elaboratory' at Trinity College, Cambridge, 229
Berengarius, Jacobus, dissection of corpses by, 4; driven from Bologna retires to Ferrara, 5
Birds, René de Reaumur on the digestion of, 207, 208
Black, Joseph, *Dissertatio de humore acido a cibo orto* of, 230; Professor of Chemistry at Glasgow and Edinburgh, *ib.*; experiments on magnesia alba, etc., *ib.*; the *Treatise of Chemistry* of, 231–234
Blas, term used by van Helmont, 130, 134, 141
Boerhaave, Hermann, birth, 198; early years at Leyden; Doctor of Philosophy, 198; of Medicine; appointed to the Chair of Medicine at Leyden, 199; death, 200; the *Institutiones medicae* of, 201; the *Elements of Chemistry* of, 225
Borelli, Giovanni Alphonso, birth, 61; studies mathematics at Rome; accepts the Chair of Mathematics

at Messina; goes to Florence to hear Galileo; returns to Messina; publishes his first work, an account of the Pestilence in Sicily, *ib.*; accepts the Chair of Mathematics at Pisa; a self-taught man, 62; friendship with Malpighi, *ib.*; becomes estranged from him; publication of his *Euclides restitutus*, 63; *De vi percussionis*; at work at the *De motu animalium*; publishes his treatise on 'The natural movements depending on gravity,' *ib.*; leaves Pisa and returns to Messina; goes into exile at Rome, 64; investigates an eruption of Etna, *ib.*; Christina, daughter of Gustavus Adolphus, takes him under her protection, 64, 65; dedicates his work on animal motion to her, 64; robbed by his servant; takes up his abode among the Society of the Scholae Piae of San Pantaleone; death, *ib.*; publication of *De motu animalium*, 65; account of the book, 65–67; on muscular contraction, 67–73; on the circulation, 74–78; on the structure of glands, 79–80; on the secretion of urine, *ib.*; on the physiology of nerves, 81; makes the friendship of Malpighi at Pisa, 87; his character contrasted with that of Malpighi, *ib.*, 88; contrasted with Franc. Sylvius, 158, 159; on gastric digestion, 163, 164; on respiration, 174–177; on muscular contraction and nervous action, 279–282
Bossuet, J. B., endeavours to convert Stensen to the Catholic religion, 105
Boyle, Hon. Robert, pneumatic machine of, 176, 177
Brunner, J. C. von, birth; graduates at Strassburg; occupies the Chair of Medicine in Heidelberg; Court Physician at Düsseldorf; death; publishes *Experimenta nova circa pancreas*; and *Dissertatio de glandulis duodeni*, 161; Brunner's glands, 162; experiment on the removal of the spleen and pancreas, 162, 163

Caesalpinus, Andreas, birth; Professor of Medicine at Pisa; Professor at the Sapienza University; Physician to Pope Clement VIII, 31; passion

Milton Keynes UK
Ingram Content Group UK Ltd.
UKHW041521181024
449640UK00009B/124